Praise for Help Your Teenager Beat an Eating Disorder

"Drs. Lock and Le Grange are two of the foremost experts in the eating disorders field. The third edition of this book condenses what the authors have learned over decades of working with the families of people with eating disorders—and puts it in a format parents can use."

—Janet Treasure, PhD, FRCP, FRCPsych,
Centre for Research in Eating Disorders,
Kings College London, United Kingdom

"This book is essential reading for any parent or family member of a teen with an eating disorder. It's especially useful for those who have been told to 'not be the food police' or that they have no role in helping support a loved one with an eating disorder. It offers practical advice for how to help, along with something just as important: hope."

—Harriet Brown, author of *Brave Girl Eating:
A Family's Struggle with Anorexia*

"This book is invaluable for parents, who often feel disempowered and blamed when their child has an eating disorder. It uses straightforward language and realistic, pragmatic examples. The third edition has been updated to incorporate the latest research and incredibly useful practical strategies. I highly recommend this book to all parents of children with eating disorders."

—Kerri Boutelle, PhD, Professor of Pediatrics,
Public Health, and Psychiatry,
University of California, San Diego

"The updated third edition of this seminal guide incorporates recent advances in eating disorders research and clinical practice, highlighting the evolving nature of the field and the authors' commitment to providing respectful, accurate parent education at each step."

—Katharine L. Loeb, PhD, Chicago Center
for Evidence Based Treatment

"There are many red flags that parents should recognize when it comes to their adolescent daughter or son's eating habits, and this intelligent book points them out clearly and concisely."
—*Publishers Weekly*

"The book is of high quality and would be of help to any family facing this difficult situation."
—*Doody's Review Service*

Help Your Teenager Beat an Eating Disorder

Also from James Lock and Daniel Le Grange

FOR PROFESSIONALS

Adolescent-Focused Therapy for Anorexia Nervosa:
A Developmental Approach
James Lock

Eating Disorders in Children and Adolescents:
A Clinical Handbook
Edited by Daniel Le Grange and James Lock

Treating Bulimia in Adolescents: A Family-Based Approach
Daniel Le Grange and James Lock

Treatment Manual for Anorexia Nervosa:
A Family-Based Approach, Third Edition
James Lock and Daniel Le Grange

Help Your Teenager Beat an Eating Disorder

THIRD EDITION

James Lock, MD, PhD
Daniel Le Grange, PhD

THE GUILFORD PRESS
New York   London

Copyright © 2025 The Guilford Press
A Division of Guilford Publications, Inc.
www.guilford.com

All rights reserved

The information in this volume is not intended as a substitute for consultation with healthcare professionals. Each individual's health concerns should be evaluated by a qualified professional.

No part of this book may be reproduced, translated, stored in a retrieval system, or transmitted, in any form or by any means, electronic, mechanical, photocopying, microfilming, recording, or otherwise, without written permission from the publisher.

Printed in the United States of America

This book is printed on acid-free paper.

For product and safety concerns within the EU, please contact GPSR@taylorandfrancis.com, Taylor & Francis Verlag GmbH, Kaufingerstraße 24, 80331 München, Germany.

Last digit is print number: 9 8 7 6 5 4 3 2 1

Library of Congress Cataloging-in-Publication Data is available from the publisher.

ISBN 978-1-4625-5712-7 (paperback) — ISBN 978-1-4625-5781-3 (hardcover)

To my children
—J. L.

To the memory of my mother and father
—D. L. G.

We would like to thank all the many patients and families with whom we have worked over the years for helping us learn how best to help them.

Contents

	Introduction	1
PART I	**GETTING STARTED** First Steps toward Helping Your Child with an Eating Disorder	
Chapter 1	Act Now	13
Chapter 2	Get Together	38
Chapter 3	Don't Waste Time on "Why"	61
PART II	**UNDERSTANDING EATING DISORDERS**	
Chapter 4	Know What You're Dealing With *The Complexity of Eating Disorders*	83
Chapter 5	Get Into Your Child's Head *The Distorted Thinking Behind Your Teenager's Behavior*	104

Chapter 6	**Understand Your Options** *What the Research Says about the Best Ways to Treat Anorexia Nervosa, Bulimia Nervosa, Binge-Eating Disorder, and Avoidant/Restrictive Food Intake Disorder*	128

PART III   MAKING TREATMENT WORK
How to Solve Everyday Problems
to Help Your Child Recover

Chapter 7	**Taking Charge of Change** *How to Apply Family-Based Treatment to Help with Eating Disorders*	153
Chapter 8	**Playing a Supporting Role** *Other Ways You Can Be a Part of Your Child's Recovery*	195
Chapter 9	**Harnessing the Power of Unity** *How to Stay on the Same Page in Your Fight against Eating Disorders*	222
Chapter 10	**Staying Empowered and Informed** *How to Work with Professionals Who Are Trying to Help Your Child*	245

Resources	263
Further Reading	271
Index	274
About the Authors	286

Introduction

When your children are sick, you don't just bring them home from the doctor's office or hospital and leave them to their own defenses. If it's the flu, the child needs fluids and rest and medicine to bring the fever down. If it's an allergy, someone needs to check package labels to make sure the allergen isn't included in a food. If your child has asthma, you make sure the inhaler is available and watch vigilantly for signs of an attack. And if your child has a very serious illness, like cancer or heart disease, you don't just expect it to get better on its own.

Someone needs to be there when the doctor isn't. That person is you. Parents are an integral part of the treatment of their children for every illness you can think of. Why, then, should it be different for eating disorders?

It shouldn't. Eating disorders are extremely serious illnesses that can threaten your child's very survival. By their nature, they are self-perpetuating and insidious. That's why a significant proportion of teenagers and adults who have eating disorders end up in the hospital at some point during the course of their illness: They need the constant, consistent vigilance of a team of professionals to ensure that they return to normal weight and normal eating habits.

The trouble is what happens when they get home. Many treatment programs for eating disorders still advocate keeping parents out of their teenager's care for a variety of reasons that we explain in this book. The consequence is often a relapse. When an eating disorder still has a hold on a teenager, leaving the child to manage it on her own once she's at home just gives the eating disorder a chance to slip through the flimsy defenses of self-care and send her on a downward spiral toward physical and psychological damage once more.

For more than three decades we have watched adolescents and their parents struggle with this horrible cycle of getting better and then getting worse again. Most of those who come to our offices arrive feeling anxious about their child's bewildering condition and overwhelmed or even defeated by this strange illness. Numerous parents have already been told by other professionals to stay on the sidelines or they will "make things worse." Many are confused in general, not quite knowing whether their child really has an eating disorder, or what precisely an eating disorder is, or what they should do about it.

We wrote this book to clear up misconceptions that we have found—and that the research is beginning to reveal—only make it harder for adolescents to recover from eating disorders: that you are to blame for the problem, that your child needs to be treated without any input or involvement (aka "interference") by you, that you need to leave diagnosis and treatment to the professionals in a way you would never agree to if your child had cancer or a heart problem, or even a broken bone. This book therefore has one simple purpose: to help you understand eating disorders and their insidious nature and to show you how you can help your child in "plugging those tiny cracks" where the eating disorder keeps slipping into his life.

That doesn't mean this book is a "self-help" manual. Eating disorders are very serious illnesses, and there is only preliminary evidence that family self-help approaches are sufficient by themselves for adolescents and their families. Instead, this book is intended to provide straight answers and hard facts about eating disorders based on the available research evidence and our own extensive clinical experience. Its goal is to offer you a perspective that is gaining more and more evidence to support it: that you have a central role to play in helping your child recover. We believe, in fact, that you are key to your teenager's return to health. This applies whether you are just considering having your child evaluated by a doctor or your child has undergone several other treatments in the past and has not yet conquered this illness. You are certainly in the best possible position to take action fast, before an eating disorder has an opportunity to do serious damage to your child's health. The research shows that when anorexia nervosa and bulimia nervosa are treated early, there is a better chance of full recovery. It is still too soon to know if early intervention will lead to better outcomes in those children with avoidant/restrictive food intake disorder (ARFID), but it seems plausible to postulate this would likely be the case. So, if nothing else, we hope this book moves you to take your child's eating disorder seriously and get help *now*. Ideally, the book will help you go further than that: It should help you establish a foundation on which you and the clinicians you work with can build a successful partnership in defeating the disorder that has overtaken your child. We hope to demystify eating disorders, and at the same time we encourage you to consider how you can help with the problems that these disorders are causing for your child and family.

The parents who come to our offices usually arrive believing they *shouldn't* be involved or feeling ineffective in helping with their child's eating disorder. This message typically comes from an external source, because few parents would subscribe instinctively to "staying out of it" if their child had any other serious illness. Therefore, this book may appear at first to be taking a radical stance. We hope you'll realize that is not the case when you read the data in Chapter 6 and elsewhere, which show that parents' participation in treatment can make an enormous positive contribution to the recovery of an adolescent with an eating disorder. Regardless of the cause, specific eating disorder diagnosis, or treatment type, we argue in this book that you not only can but should be involved. This book will help you figure out how.

The approach we mostly use in our own treatment centers, which is now the approach with the largest evidence of effectiveness, is called *family-based treatment* (FBT). The concept behind this treatment is derived from decades of family work involving anorexia at the Child Guidance Resource Center in Philadelphia, and the Maudsley

Hospital in London, in the 1970s and 1980s. This seminal work illustrates the importance of parents' involvement and support in finding solutions to the dilemmas faced by their adolescents with eating disorders. This perspective stands in stark contrast to approaches that blame parents and exclude them from treatment. Over the past 30 years, systematic delivery and empirical research have demonstrated the effectiveness of FBT for eating disorders in youth.

The fact that this book is for parents in the first place sets it apart from many books on eating disorders. When this book was first published, most of these books in print were directed at adults or teenagers themselves who were ill, which left a big gap in sources of information for parents. That's why we initially crafted this book to answer the questions that parents had brought to us over many years of our practice and still bring to us—everything from "Am I to blame?" to "What do I do when he disappears after a meal and I know he is going to throw it all up?," "Just how do we get her to eat a healthy meal again when she won't let us?," "Shouldn't she be on some medication as well?," and "I don't understand this illness; isn't the solution straightforward—you eat, and that's that?"

We have been gathering answers to these questions, separately and together, for a combined total of more than 60 years as clinician–researchers (meaning that we see patients and we also conduct research studies) treating adolescents with eating disorders at academic medical centers. Eating disorders are not rare: Each of us has seen hundreds of patients and their parents, and it is likely that you as parents know someone who has had an eating disorder. We have treated patients in inpatient settings, group programs, and individual and family therapies. We have spent our academic careers exploring how better to help adolescents with eating disorders, and this book is an important part of that effort.

Each chapter in this newest edition has been substantially revised, providing updates on clinical factors and treatment research related to eating disorders in youth. We've streamlined the examples and added new ones related to key interventions and concepts discussed. Happily, since the publication of the second edition of this book, research on the treatment of eating disorders in children and adolescents has made advances, particularly in documenting the effectiveness and efficiency of family interventions for these disorders. We also describe the impact, which is mostly positive, of the revisions in the diagnostic system used to categorize mental disorders of child and adolescent eating disorders. The fifth edition of the American Psychiatric Association's *Diagnostic and Statistical Manual of Mental Disorders* (DSM-5) better took into account developmental issues related to eating disorders, including making the requirements for the diagnosis of bulimia and anorexia less stringent and adding new eating disorder diagnoses, including binge-eating disorder and ARFID. We discuss what we know about how these disorders present and current approaches to treating these disorders that are under investigation.

A particular issue that has struck us in a very meaningful way is just how resourceful parents usually are and what a great resource they are when they are brought into the treatment process. We strongly believe that if parents can be helped to get a better understanding of eating disorders and to take definite early steps to intervene in these problems in a constructive way, many lives will be improved and some lives actually saved.

Both of us have worked as clinicians and researchers in academic medical settings for the past three decades. Although we started this work in different parts of the world, our mutual interest in the treatment of adolescents with eating disorders has brought us together in our thinking about how best to do what we do on a daily basis in our respective practices. This has led to a rich and productive collaboration that started in 1998 when we jointly wrote our first book, a manual for clinicians who treat adolescents with anorexia nervosa. Since then we have conducted numerous workshops about this treatment throughout the world. We discuss our difficult cases with each other, we present our research findings at professional meetings, and we continue to collaborate on ongoing and new clinical treatment studies. Since the publication of the first and second editions of this volume, we have been pleased that increased attention to the role of parents in helping their children with eating disorders has led to the founding of several parent organizations (Families Empowered and Supporting Treatment of Eating Disorders, or FEAST, as an example) that are strong advocates for increased awareness of the role of parents in helping their children, demanding better clinical services for eating disorders and promoting new research efforts to learn more about how to help children and adolescents with eating disorders. Furthermore, we are told daily that eating disorder treatment programs around the world use this book to educate families about their role in helping their children with these problems. Therefore, we are thrilled that this book has been translated into Portuguese, Japanese, Dutch, Polish, Italian, Mandarin, Spanish, and Russian. Throughout all this work with adolescents and their parents, we are reminded every day of the real value of parents' contributions to the treatment process. It is this collective experience of treating teenagers with eating disorders, engaging their parents in this process, and researching and writing about these experiences in academic journals that continues to inspire us to involve parents in the process through writing this book.

HOW TO USE THIS BOOK

This book is divided into three parts. The titles for the chapters were chosen carefully to draw your attention to the urgency of the matter, to highlight the most salient aspects of eating disorders, and then, with this knowledge, to help you respond to your child's illness in the best possible way. If our use of imperatives such as "Act Now," "Get Together," and "Don't Waste Time" seems powerful, it's intended to get your attention. It's human nature to hope that a health problem will go away on its own, but to postpone seeking help for your child can be extremely dangerous. Sadly, treatment approaches that rob you of your rightful role as guardian of your child's health only encourage you to let others make critical decisions about what to do and when.

In Part I of this book, we focus on *why* you need to take action now if your child has symptoms of an eating disorder. We discuss why eating disorders are serious problems, and why you must act together as parents to get treatment started and worry less about "why" this problem developed and more about "how" to get it eradicated. Dealing with eating disorders effectively always requires you to perceive your child's eating disorder as an urgent matter that needs your prompt attention. In fact, *urgent* is the byword for Part I. It's worth repeating what we said earlier: If your child has signs of an eating disorder, it's urgent that your child gets help, and it's you, the parents, who are in the best possible position to see that your child gets this help.

Part II provides you with more "nuts and bolts" about eating disorders. Eating disorders can be very confusing to doctors, parents, and sufferers alike. Therefore, it's important for you to know what you're up against, perhaps even more so than with many other types of illness. The purpose of this section of the book is to help you appreciate the complexities of these illnesses. We discuss the various types of eating disorders, particularly anorexia nervosa, bulimia nervosa, binge-eating disorder, and ARFID, as well as how starvation and binge eating and purging can lead to severe medical problems. You will find that we often discuss eating disorders as if they were entities independent of your child. We do this to stress our view that eating disorders are illnesses and not willful choices being made by your child to oppose you. Next we illustrate how a young person with an eating disorder thinks. The distortions common to such thought processes are illustrated to underscore the need for treatment. They can also help you separate the illness from the child so that you can remain supportive of your child, who is, after all, suffering from real distortions about experiences of the body, and thoughts and beliefs about food and weight. We end this part with information about the main treatment approaches for eating disorders and the evidence available for their effectiveness so that you'll have a good scientific understanding of what may help your child and what may not.

Part III is designed to help you tackle the practical problems you will face in trying to get and use help for your child's eating disorder. We illustrate various ways that parents can be involved in each of the known major treatments for eating disorders, even if the form of treatment may appear to discourage parental involvement. We also offer tips to help you confront the cultural forces that contribute to disordered thinking about food and weight. Most important, though, is the partnership that we mentioned earlier. To seal up those cracks that your child's eating disorder will do its best to slip through, the entire treatment team needs to establish a united front to fight the illness. This means that parents—or you and any other adults who are invested in helping your child recover—need to be "on the same page" in dealing with the illness at all times. It means that you also need to find a way to form a fruitful alliance with the professionals on your treatment team. Consequently, this part includes chapters that help you stave off the eating disorder's efforts to "divide and conquer" and help you stand your ground constructively when you have disagreements with the experts who are trying to cure your teenage son or daughter.

WHAT YOU WILL LEARN FROM THIS BOOK

After you have read this book, we hope you will feel confident that you have a role in helping your child recover from an eating disorder. You should know the ways in which eating disorders develop and when to get worried as your child's normal concerns about her body, food, eating, and exercise become increasingly abnormal. You will know the medical problems that can and will develop if your child's eating disorder isn't treated effectively. You will know what to expect when you have your child evaluated and what kinds of treatments are likely to be offered. You will learn that parental involvement can take many forms, such as helping your child eat at home, supporting individual therapy for your child when needed, monitoring binge-eating and purging episodes, and participating in treatments that enhance your child's interpersonal capacities and roles.

We also hope that after reading this book you will be certain that there is help for your child with an eating disorder and that the resources we provide at the conclusion will be helpful to you in determining where to go for this assistance.

A NOTE FROM THE AUTHORS

This book is not intended as a self-help guide, nor is it intended in any way to substitute for the advice of a physician or therapist.

Introduction

Moreover, research into eating disorders, their causes, and the best treatments is ongoing; to stay abreast of advances in the field, consult reliable sources such as those listed in the Resources and Further Reading sections.

This book is aimed at helping parents with children and adolescents, and transition-age youth (18–25 years old).

Eating disorders increasingly affect all genders, although anorexia and bulimia nervosa are more common in girls. That said, all statements in this book, unless otherwise noted, apply to all genders. To emphasize this point, we vary pronouns in examples throughout the text. We also include many examples of children with eating disorders, which are thoroughly disguised to protect privacy or presented as composites of real clinical cases.

PART I

GETTING STARTED

First Steps toward Helping
Your Child with an Eating Disorder

CHAPTER 1

Act Now

You don't know what to do.

Thirteen-year-old Sheila has been losing weight for 6 months. At first you thought it was normal teenage dieting. But she's too thin now. She has stopped eating with you but insists on cooking everything for the whole household. Last week she made four desserts but wouldn't eat any of them. She has a book with a list of the calories in everything most of us eat, but she doesn't need it anymore because she knows it by heart. Besides, at present, she eats only three things: raw vegetables, tofu, and dry cereal. She's still doing well in school. Her straight As, though, seem more of a burden than a source of accomplishment to her. When she isn't studying, she's going for a run or doing sit-ups. She ignores calls from her friends and seems more and more depressed. When you try to encourage her to eat, she fumes and says it's none of your business. She insists she's fine.

You don't know what to do.

You caught 17-year-old Donna throwing up. She said she was sick. But it wasn't the first time. You have heard her before. Always heading off to the bathroom after every meal. She says it was nothing—she only had an upset stomach. You've noticed she hardly eats breakfast or lunch, but when you come home in the evening, lots of food is gone from the pantry, especially cookies, potato chips, and bread. You've had to go to the store midweek to restock. One of her friends told you she is worried about Donna. You are too.

You don't know what to do.

Tom used to be a great high school diver. He's too weak now to perform his toughest dives. He consumes only protein bars and fruit drinks. He is constantly exercising to get perfect abdominal muscles, but you can see his ribs. He says he's still too fat. Where there used to be muscle, there's mostly bone and skin now. At first his coach complimented Tom on his weight loss because it had improved his dive entries. Now the coach has called you and suggested Tom take a leave from the team. Tom's best friend called him "skeleton" to tease him, but you know he's worried too.

You don't know what to do.

Every morning when you go to the cupboards you find things have gone missing—usually whole bags of chips, boxes of cereal, packages of cookies. When you're cleaning Rick's room, you find empty packets stashed under the bed, crumbs on the sheets and blankets, and empty food containers in the trash bin. You are hesitant to say anything because you don't want to make a big deal of his eating, but you can't help but notice he is gaining a lot of weight and has started to not fit into his clothes. He is also spending less time with friends and no longer plays pickup basketball with them. He says he's bored with the game, but he seems to get winded even climbing the stairs to his room.

You don't know what to do.

Timothy has always been thin. He is always too busy to eat and when he says he's hungry, he only eats a few bites then says he's full and leaves the table to play on his computer. You pack his lunch, but more often than not when he comes home from school it is only partially eaten at best. He says he forgot or didn't have time to eat. This has been going on for his whole life and his pediatrician has been saying he'll grow out of it, but all his friends are starting to grow taller and he's not showing any signs of puberty. He doesn't seem concerned about it, but you notice he is not keeping up with the others on his soccer team as well as he used to, needing more breaks and not able to run as fast.

You don't know what to do. *Should* you do something?

This is the first problem you face if you're concerned that your son or daughter may have an eating disorder. You know most eating problems in children are transient. You remember lots of struggles over junk food and sweets with your other children, or you've seen it in other families. Many children commonly go through periods of being picky eaters, eating more than usual, eating less than usual, and even complaining about upset stomachs or having periods of mild digestive problems and constipation. You've asked other parents and relatives about these types of behaviors and learned that, although usually short-lived, eating problems are nearly universal. As children enter puberty, many, especially girls, are very much interested in their appearance and weight and may try dieting or other weight-loss strategies. You expect this because you know it's normal to become more concerned about appearance in the teenage years and because you've known your son's or daughter's friends to express similar thoughts and engage in the same types of behavior. You don't want to create a problem where there isn't one.

How do you know if there's a real problem?

If you think your child's thoughts and behaviors resemble those of Sheila, Donna, Tom, Rick, or Timothy, however, it's time to take action to help. Left untreated, eating disorders can lead to chronic health problems, depression, and even death. With the severe weight loss associated with anorexia nervosa, for example, starvation leads to lower body temperature, decreased blood pressure, and decreased heart rate, as well as rough and dry skin, loss of hair, cessation of menstruation in young women, and osteoporosis. Because the body isn't being fed, it turns to muscle for fuel. This causes weakness, fatigue, and, in particular, decreased cardiac mass (the heart being a large muscle in the body), which can prompt dangerous changes in heart rhythm and may thereby cause cardiac failure and death. Over time, the risk of death as a result of the complications of anorexia is estimated at 6–15%. This mortality rate is the highest for any psychiatric disease.

For bulimia nervosa, the risk for death appears to be lower, but there still are risks of severe medical complications. One of the most common of these complications is depletion of potassium (hypokalemia), which results from loss of body stores of this essential electrolyte due to purging stomach contents. Without potassium, which is required for many basic physical processes but is very important for muscle contraction, cardiac arrhythmias are possible, leading to cardiac arrest and death. In addition, with chronic vomiting, the linings of the esophagus and stomach can become eroded, causing bleeding, ulcers, erosion of tooth enamel, and even death if the bleeding cannot be stopped. Chronic use of laxatives and purgatives leads to intestinal problems, including pain and severe and unremitting constipation. Both vomiting and the use of laxatives lead to severe depletion of water from the body (dehydration), which can cause low and changing blood pressure, increasing the likelihood of fainting and falls.

For binge-eating disorder, the medical risks include obesity, hypertension, and diabetes. These problems are potentially lifelong and in many cases lead to a decreased quality of life, including challenges with mobility, travel, and relationships. The need for surgical intervention to address joint problems also increases. Hypertension and diabetes increase the risk of cardiac problems and early mortality.

The specific medical risks associated with avoidant/restrictive food intake disorder vary depending on the specific type of symptoms, their duration, and the age of the child. For those who primarily present with lack of interest in eating, low appetite, or fear of choking or vomiting, leading to weight loss or failure to gain weight appropriate for age, height, or gender, many of the medical risks are identical to those associated with malnutrition in anorexia nervosa—cardiac instability, bone loss, and in severe cases, death. If the child is entering puberty, there is a risk of short stature and related hormonal insufficiencies. In children who are highly selective in the range of foods they eat but consume enough to be in the normal weight range, medical problems can still occur, particularly related to nutritional insufficiencies.

We discuss these complications in more detail in Chapter 4. By now, though, you can undoubtedly see that eating disorders have serious health consequences. To be complacent in the face of a possible eating disorder is the greatest risk a parent can take in the battle to prevent such serious problems from developing.

WHAT DOES AN EATING DISORDER LOOK LIKE AS IT DEVELOPS?

If you're to catch a problem before it becomes an eating disorder, you have to know what to look for over time. Sheila, Donna, Tom, Rick, and Timothy's problems did not develop in a day. Like most eating disorders, their problems developed gradually and sometimes in secret. If you understand the path by which more typical, temporary eating problems and weight concerns can become real eating disorders, you can get a sense of where your own child is on that trajectory.

Extreme Dieting: The Path to Anorexia Nervosa

> Fourteen-year-old Rosa has always been a terrific child. Her parents said she had spoiled them because she was always so easy, independent, reliable, and mature. That's why they were so shocked by her recent weight loss. She had never shown the slightest sign of emotional problems. She was an honor student, swim team champ, and popular at school. She had never been overweight; in fact, she'd always been on the thin side.
>
> The problems seemed to begin during the summer before ninth grade. Rosa had been on the summer swim team. It was the first time her parents noticed that she wanted to stay longer

to swim after practice. She wanted to get fitter, she said, so she could be a starter on both the breaststroke and freestyle teams. At the same time, she started a vegetarian diet. She felt it was cruel to eat animals, and besides, she didn't need fat in her diet when she was trying to be healthier. At first her parents understood and supported her efforts at self-improvement as Rosa seemed happy and confident.

Then Rosa attended the special 3-week swim camp for the summer team located in another part of the state. She left in the middle of July and returned at the end of the first week of August. When her parents picked her up at the bus, they were startled, almost frightened by how thin Rosa had become. They didn't say anything right away. They were just glad to have their daughter home. They surmised that the food hadn't been too good at the camp, and Rosa implied as much. They didn't have good vegetarian choices, she said, and she was very active. She had made both teams as a starter.

And then school began. The ninth grade was a transitional year for Rosa. Students from three middle schools were combined in a single high school, so there were many new kids in her class. Her parents noticed that Rosa seemed more preoccupied and worried about schoolwork, but they thought this was to be expected when starting high school. Rosa's day began at 5:00 A.M. with swim practice for 2 hours before school. She then attended classes for the day and reported for another swim practice from 5:00 to 7:00 P.M. Rosa arrived home after the family had already eaten. She studied until 11:00 P.M.

Out of sight of her parents, Rosa had developed a highly limited eating pattern. She allowed herself one cup of orange juice before morning practice. She told her mother she had a bagel and cream cheese at school with milk after practice, but in reality, she ate half a dry bagel and drank water. The lunch her mother carefully prepared for her was thrown away each day. Again before afternoon practice, she would drink a glass of orange juice. Because she came home after the family had eaten, her parents didn't know how much she had for dinner. Usually she had a carefully weighed slice of tofu, a few carrots, and an apple.

Her parents grew increasingly alarmed at Rosa's continued weight loss. The coach of the swim team called to ask what was wrong with Rosa. She was afraid that Rosa might have an eating disorder. Her parents made an appointment with her pediatrician, which took some time to set up. When they arrived, the pediatrician said that Rosa was too thin, and Rosa promised to eat more. Unfortunately, she did not. Her parents tried to intervene, but she easily became angry when they talked to her about eating, and they hated to confront her.

Rosa became too weak to swim and was taken off the swim team. At school, she was more and more isolated, and her friends stopped talking to her because they were afraid to ask her what was wrong. She became tearful and moody at home. She was so thin now that none of her clothes fit, even though they had been purchased only a month before, when school began. She was always cold; she wore sweaters and was constantly turning up the heat while the rest of the family sweltered. Her worried parents thought she was depressed and sought help from a psychiatrist.

Although anorexia nervosa usually starts in early adolescence, typically at 13–14 years, it is not uncommon to see children between the ages of 8 and 11 develop this eating disorder. Anorexia usually begins with an episode of dieting that gradually leads to life-threatening starvation. At times some identifiable precipitating event triggers the dieting process. Maybe the child is teased about her weight, or her friends start dieting. Or perhaps she sees her parents dieting. Some girls start dieting at the onset of menses, when they make the transition to a new school or level in school, or when they begin dating. The illness of a parent may also trigger dieting. It's important to understand that these events often start the dieting process, but that does not mean these triggers are the causes of anorexia nervosa. It is dieting that usually appears to be the starting point for anorexia nervosa.

Teens diet for a number of reasons. Sheila says she began dieting to become a healthier person, whereas Tom's dieting was initially designed to improve his diving. Most teenagers report that dieting began because of a wish to lose weight, eat healthier, or improve performance in a sport. A few adolescents begin consuming fewer calories in the service of being "good," as they define it, using an ascetic formulation along the lines of "the less you consume, the better you are."

All these motivations to diet share some features. For example, each implies some notion of self-improvement, in particular improvements that are concrete and outward and thus noticeable by others—to look better, perform better, be healthier. However, there are differences among these motivations for dieting as well. The emphasis on a thin appearance suggests a connection with social norms of beauty, whereas improvement in performance of a sport, in health, or in morality is related more directly to perfectionism, drive, and ambition. These latter qualities appear to be common personality features in children who develop eating disorders.

Regardless of motivation, dieting usually begins informally. The child may start by cutting out desserts and snacks, but over time, meats and other proteins, fats, and sugars are eliminated too. Once food choices are narrowed, dieting efforts are typically focused on lowering the quantities of food consumed even within this limited range of options. Often detailed calorie counting, exact measuring, and elaborate preparation of foods become the rule. At this point, adolescents may attempt to remove themselves from the company of others while eating, prepare meals independently of others, and sometimes cook elaborate meals and desserts for others without eating the food themselves.

Alongside this extreme food restriction, a schedule of increased exercise is often employed to ensure continued weight loss. At this point, whatever weight goals might have been set initially have typically been long surpassed, and the goal of weight loss in itself is firmly established. Sometimes self-induced vomiting or diet pill and laxative use may begin in an attempt to purge the small portions consumed.

For a child on the path to an eating disorder, on the one hand, eating is often associated with guilt, anxiety, and anger. Not eating, on the other hand, is associated with feelings of accomplishment, power, and strength. Paradoxically, with increased weight loss, hunger cues are diminished, making the process of continued food restriction easier. Nonetheless, most teens with anorexia are still extraordinarily preoccupied with food. Some will visit supermarkets and bakeries to look at and smell the food, but abstain from eating it. Parents may notice unusual food rituals beginning to develop, such as eating only out of certain bowls or plates, weighing and measuring foods precisely, using chopsticks, and so forth. The period of time over which this cascade of events takes place is variable, but it can be as short as 4–6 weeks or as long as a year or more. At some point during this process, in girls who have begun menses, menstruation likely ceases.

In the 2013 iteration of the American Psychiatric Association's *Diagnostic and Statistical Manual of Mental Disorders*, DSM-5, another form of anorexia nervosa was described as "atypical anorexia nervosa," or more precisely, other specified feeding or eating disorders (OSFED). The main difference between typical and atypical anorexia nervosa is that the weight of the individual with atypical anorexia nervosa is not low according to typical height and weight calculations. Instead, the young person with atypical anorexia nervosa has usually started off at a higher weight than average, but has lost significant weight rapidly and with all the associated disordered cognitions and behaviors typical of anorexia nervosa. They are just as "lost" in anorexic thoughts and are just as behaviorally compulsive around eating and exercise, and they can become just as seriously medically ill as those with typical anorexia nervosa. When we speak of anorexia nervosa in this book, we are including under that rubric atypical anorexia nervosa as well because other than degree of weight loss, these disorders are very similar.

Failed Dieting and Overeating: The Path to Bulimia Nervosa

Sixteen-year-old Jasmine had always set high standards for herself. She wanted to be the best at everything. She worked hard at school and got good grades. She was generally well liked, though she always worried about who her friends were. She had worried about her weight for as long as she could remember and first began trying to lose weight when she went on a liquid diet with her mother when she was in fifth grade. She herself was never teased for being overweight, but she had seen other girls and boys teased when she was a child and was worried that she too would be teased. The diets she tried never made any difference. She lost a few pounds but then gained the weight back.

For the junior prom Jasmine decided she wanted to look great. She had a boyfriend, her first, and she wanted him to find her beautiful. That meant *thin*. Her boyfriend had never commented on her weight, but Jasmine was sure it was just because he was too nice to say anything. She knew she was too fat. She was determined to lose 15 pounds before the prom.

She began skipping breakfast altogether, and lunch as well. She would then go to the gym after school and exercise for 2 hours. She found some over-the-counter diet pills and drank lots of coffee, all in an effort to keep herself from being so hungry. Still, she woke up at night feeling hungry. But she stuck with her routine and lost 15 pounds for the prom. Everyone told her how wonderful she looked, and her boyfriend seemed happy with her appearance too. All her friends congratulated her on her diet and wanted to know how she did it.

After the prom Jasmine tried to keep her diet plan going, but it became harder and harder to do. She would come home from school and be too tired to go to the gym. When she missed her workout, she was certain she would gain weight, so she tried to eat even less the next day. However, she began to be so hungry that she couldn't stop herself from eating. One day after school when no one else was home, Jasmine was so hungry that she ate a box of cookies. She went to the gym and tried to "exercise the calories away," but there were too many and she was too tired. The same thing happened the next day. This time Jasmine was so upset she decided to try to throw up the cookies. She had promised herself that she would never do this, but she couldn't stand the worry about gaining weight. She would throw up just this once.

Jasmine tried to follow her own injunction, and sometimes she succeeded, but at least once or twice a week she failed and overate so much that she felt she had to purge. Slowly, week by week, she got into a pattern of eating very little and then binge eating in the afternoon, followed by purging. On days she found she couldn't vomit, she took some of her mother's laxatives to relieve her fears about gaining weight.

During this time, Jasmine's weight had gradually increased despite her efforts to diet, using diet pills and laxatives, and vomiting. Jasmine was increasingly despondent. Her boyfriend broke up with her because she stopped wanting to get together with him. She felt too ashamed of her weight to see him. In addition, she was afraid to go out with him because she might have to eat something and that would start her overeating.

Jasmine's mother hadn't suspected anything until one day she heard Jasmine throwing up in the shower. She asked her what was wrong, and Jasmine confessed to throwing up purposely, but only that one time. Still, her mother remained concerned and noticed that Jasmine had taken some laxatives from the medicine cabinet. Again, Jasmine denied she used them to lose weight, claiming she had done so because she was constipated. Finally, the mother of one of Jasmine's girlfriends called Jasmine's mother to tell her that her daughter had caught Jasmine throwing up at school. Jasmine's mother now tried to find help.

Binge-eating episodes and purging usually begin a little later than the extreme dieting of anorexia nervosa. Still, adolescents who binge eat and purge often report long histories of preoccupation with weight. Some say they remember worrying about their weight as early as kindergarten. Some were mildly to moderately obese during early childhood and remember being teased. Often these adolescents have experimented with a variety of diets for brief periods, only to abandon such efforts. Many report that in response to severe dieting and fasting behaviors, they develop an urge to overeat and feel increasingly out of control when eating. Once they've overeaten, they feel guilty and anxious and, as a result, seek ways to relieve themselves of their fear of gaining weight. This leads to purging in its various forms. Most often purging is accomplished through vomiting, but it can also include the use of laxatives, diuretics, and compensatory exercise.

Adolescents with bulimia nervosa, like their adult counterparts, report that to a great degree their self-worth depends on feeling satisfied with their weight and appearance. Often these adolescents report that they eat very little breakfast or lunch, but that upon returning to their homes after school, they binge. This is a time when there is usually little parental supervision and the binge eating can occur secretly. In addition, binge eating can become a way to cope with feelings of loneliness, boredom, and anxiety. Alternately, some adolescents report nighttime binge eating, another time when they are less likely to be observed.

Most adolescents, like adults, with bulimia nervosa report intense feelings of shame about these behaviors. As the disorder becomes more entrenched, teens begin to organize their lives around the management of binge eating and the compensatory activities related to it. They become more irritable and withdraw from friends and families. Often their schoolwork declines. They also report increasingly depressed moods. Once these altered patterns of eating are firmly established and extend their hold on the adolescent, binge eating and purging become a convenient way to avoid other problems and may be increasingly incorporated into the adolescent's coping strategies. These factors combine to make bulimia nervosa surprisingly resistant to change, even when someone is motivated to make such an effort. In addition, sometimes adolescents with bulimia nervosa report a history of other impulsive behaviors, such as alcohol use and shoplifting.

> Jasmine's mother took her to see a psychologist, who diagnosed her with bulimia nervosa, but Jasmine refused to return for therapy. Her mother tried to persuade her to go, but she said she could stop the behavior on her own. It appeared that this was the case, as Jasmine's mother saw no evidence of continued purging or binge eating for several months. However, her hopes were dashed when she discovered several bags of vomit and food containers in the garage. She called the psychologist again, who suggested they come in as a family to discuss how to proceed.

Using Food to Manage Emotions and Social Difficulties: The Path to Binge-Eating Disorder

> Sheiko is 18 years old and lives with her mother and younger sister. Sheiko has been worrying about her weight since she was 12 years old. In the past year or so she began to binge eat, especially when she was alone at home or late at night. Sheiko says she often feels sad or depressed because of a fight with a friend or rejection by a potential romantic partner. She tries to eat to

make herself feel better. "Guys won't like me unless I'm skinny," she says, which then makes her sad, and she thinks if she eats she will feel better. She also binges when she is lonely: "People don't like me anyway—what's the point of losing weight?" Unfortunately, after she binges she feels like a failure. "I'm weak; I don't have any self-control," she says. Sheiko is a senior in high school and hopes to go to college. She is a good student with excellent grades.

Like many adolescents with binge-eating disorder, Sheiko began having emotional difficulties some time before the onset of binge eating. She had tried to diet, but this led to overeating in response to emotional and social crises. As in Sheiko's case, the symptoms of adolescents with binge-eating disorder intensify over time and are complicated by depression, social anxiety, shame, and feelings of failure. Most adolescents with binge-eating disorder describe using food to help with their emotions, mostly negative ones like depression and anger. Sheiko's mother took her to the pediatric clinic. The pediatrician there told Sheiko she was overweight and needed to lose weight or risk developing high blood pressure or diabetes.

Low Interest in Eating, Fear of Choking or Vomiting, and Extreme Picky Eating: The Paths to Avoidant/Restrictive Food Intake Disorder

Mike had always been small for his age, had never been a good eater, and had to be made to sit at the table to finish as much as his parents could manage to get him to eat. As a result, there were many "food fights" with Mike and his parents that made mealtimes unpleasant for everyone in the family. His parents had taken Mike to his pediatrician, who encouraged them to let him be and he would grow out of it—that is until recently, when he had fallen off his growth curve. More pressure on Mike didn't help. He would just leave the table and sulk. His parents consulted a registered dietician, who suggested a meal plan, and an occupational therapist, who found no physical explanations related to swallowing or chewing to explain Mike's lack of interest in eating. Mike's parents were exhausted from fighting with him and had just about given up on trying to help him.

Children like Mike likely are born with less interest in eating—it just isn't as pleasurable or rewarding as it is to most people. This is not their fault. They are not choosing to not eat like someone with anorexia nervosa. They simply don't really enjoy it or enjoy other things more than eating. This would be fine if this disinterest had limited impact on Mike's overall health and well-being, but this is not the case for Mike. He is falling off his growth curve and is not growing as he should, and this may lead to lifelong health problems, including short stature, delayed puberty, and emotional problems related to these developments.

Kat was previously a somewhat anxious but overall healthy girl who had no difficulty eating until she choked on a piece of pizza at a family picnic. After that incident, Kat refused to eat solid foods because she was afraid of choking. At first she would still have smoothies and soft foods like pudding and oatmeal, but soon she began to refuse these too because they felt "thick" as she swallowed and she began to spit them out. She lost weight rapidly and soon began to complain of being dizzy when she stood up and too weak to walk around or go to school. Her parents became increasingly alarmed and took her to the pediatrician, who found Kat's heart rate was below 35 beats per minute and recommended immediate hospitalization for treatment of malnutrition.

Some children who develop avoidant/restrictive food intake disorder like Kat have no history of problems with food or eating. However, in cases where there is a fear that something life-threatening could happen as a result of eating—like choking, severe allergic reaction, or vomiting—there has often been a previous event that triggered this fear. It could be something as seemingly innocuous as choking on a bite of pizza, as with Kat, or something more dramatic, like a near drowning. Regardless of the event, the child's response is to become extremely frightened about eating. It is not a fear of gaining weight or getting fat as with anorexia nervosa, but rather is a fear of some physical consequence of eating that will hurt, embarrass, or harm them. Many times these children will have an anxious temperament by history or sometimes a bona fide anxiety disorder that may increase the risk of developing avoidant/restrictive food intake disorder after a traumatic event.

DOES YOUR CHILD HAVE AN EATING DISORDER?

The first of the following lists contains items that you should be on the lookout for if you think it's possible your child is developing or has an eating disorder. If they are present, then you'll want to exercise additional vigilance to see if these warning signs are really indications that your child is developing an eating disorder that needs evaluation and treatment. The second list includes items that, if present, suggest that you need to take immediate action to have your child evaluated and treated.

Warning Signs of the Development of an Eating Disorder
- Diet books
- Evidence of visiting pro-anorexia or eating disorder websites
- Dieting behavior
- Sudden decision to become a vegetarian
- Increased picky eating, especially eating only "healthy foods"
- Always going to the bathroom immediately after eating
- Multiple showers in a day (to purge in the shower), especially directly following eating
- Unusual number of stomach flu episodes
- Skipping meals
- Large amounts of food missing

Act-Now Signs and Symptoms
- Fasting and skipping meals regularly
- Refusing to eat with the family
- Two skipped periods (in girls) in conjunction with weight loss
- Any binge-eating episodes
- Any purging episodes
- Discovery of diet pills or laxatives
- Excessive exercise (more than an hour a day) and weight loss

- Persistent and unremitting refusal to eat nondiet foods
- Refusing to allow others to prepare foods
- Extreme calorie counting or portion control (weighing and measuring food amounts)
- Refusing to eat with friends

If at this point you've determined you need to have your child evaluated for an eating disorder, you'll want to consult someone who is an expert in these problems. This usually means someone besides a pediatrician or family physician, most of whom have had little training or experience with eating disorders. Certainly all these professionals will have heard of eating disorders, and many will have had some limited experience, but most are not sure when an expert is needed, and they can unintentionally reassure parents, beyond the point at which they should, about not needing help.

This does not mean you should bypass your pediatrician or family physician on the way to an expert in eating disorders—quite the contrary. A physician can rule out other causes of your child's problems, which should get you closer to knowing whether an eating disorder is likely. Your pediatrician should be able to get an accurate weight and height for your child and perform a physical exam, including ordering basic laboratory work, that will uncover readily identifiable medical conditions that might be causing the problems you're observing—unexplained weight loss, loss of menstruation, or other physical symptoms such as lightheadedness or fainting. This examination may also reveal evidence that your child's problem is more urgent than you thought. If, for example, it turns out that your child has low blood pressure, a low heart rate, or signs of severe purging (erosion of tooth enamel, inexplicable swollen salivary glands, inexplicable weight loss), you'll know that you were right to act now. In some cases, when a teenager has developed such problems, hospitalization is necessary.

A basic medical workup for an adolescent with an eating disorder would include the following: a complete physical to check for signs of severe starvation (for example, assessment of weight relative to height, low blood pressure, low heart rate, dry skin, low body temperature), as well as tests for liver, kidney, and thyroid functioning. These examinations help assess the degree of illness and its chronicity, as well as rule out other possible organic reasons for weight loss, including diabetes, thyroid disease, or cancers. Common laboratory tests include a complete blood count; an electrocardiogram; studies of electrolytes, BUN (blood urea nitrogen), and creatinine; thyroid studies; and a test for urine specific gravity. Your pediatrician should be able to discuss the purpose of each of these tests, help you understand any unusual laboratory results, and alert you if there is any cause for immediate medical intervention.

Assuming that your child is not too sick and that another medical problem is not clearly causing the problems with eating, you will need to proceed to an evaluation by an expert in eating disorders in children and adolescents. That's why you should take advantage of this appointment with the pediatrician to find out what kind of experience the doctor has had with eating disorders. It may require a little tact and skill, but if you know the doctor fairly well, you will probably find a way to ask these important questions:

"Have you seen many adolescents with eating disorders?"
"What do you recommend in terms of treatment (both medical and psychological)?"
"Whom do you refer your patients to and why?"
"How successful do you think your patients have been with treatment?"

If your pediatrician proves not to be an expert, you can take steps to find one. We should note that pediatricians are sometimes reluctant to make referrals to such specialists because they are unsure whether changes in eating behaviors are due to emotional problems or just developmentally normal adolescent experimentation. In addition, because an adolescent with an eating disorder often denies or minimizes symptoms, physicians sometimes don't get the whole story from the adolescent. It might be helpful to go over the lists of warning signs presented earlier to encourage your pediatrician to make a referral if you have observed any of the behaviors on the "Act Now" list in your child.

A referral from your primary care physician or pediatrician often permits full insurance coverage for your child's psychiatric evaluation, so getting this referral rather than seeking an expert on your own is important for this reason as well. Scheduling such an evaluation may, unfortunately, be more complicated than it should be because of insurance processes and the limited availability of experts in eating disorders. Still, these obstacles can usually be overcome with persistence and a referral from a pediatrician specifying the need for the consultation.

Consult the Resources section at the end of this book for guidance on where to begin your search for help. One caveat, however: Many clinicians who treat adults with eating disorders are not prepared to evaluate younger patients. They are neither trained to look for the ways these younger patients' symptoms develop nor trained in ways to engage them or their parents to evaluate them effectively. There are many exceptions to this rule, of course, but the wise parent will inquire about the clinician's experience with younger patients before scheduling an appointment.

WHAT TO DO TO GET HELP

Most adolescents with eating disorders do not want help—at least initially. They see themselves as choosing to manage a problem with weight, and even if they recognize some problems with their dieting, they generally prefer to be left alone to sort it out themselves. Unfortunately, case descriptions like those you've just read make it pretty clear that many adolescents do not figure a way out soon enough to prevent serious problems from setting in. That leaves it up to parents to get the ball rolling sooner. This is easier said than done. So parents immediately face at least two problems in trying to help their child with an eating disorder: (1) how to get their child to have an evaluation for an eating disorder and (2) whom and what to look for in terms of evaluation.

How to Get Your Child to Have an Evaluation

Before you delve into the challenge of getting your child to agree to an evaluation, make sure that you and your spouse or coparent (if there are two parents) agree that there is a problem that demands an evaluation. The importance of parents working together is a major theme of this book that is discussed in more detail later, particularly in Chapter 9. But even in agreeing that there is a problem, many parents differ on what to do about it. Using the guidelines provided in our lists of warning signs may help the two of you see things the same way. And even if one parent is reluctant to move forward, the more concerned parent may have to take the lead initially to get things started. As long as the other parent doesn't manifest active opposition, this may be where some families have to start.

Once you're in agreement that your child needs a professional evaluation, it's important to let your child know you're planning to seek one. Springing the evaluation on her, which may be tempting inasmuch as you know she may resist going, can backfire because it makes it more likely that she will refuse to cooperate with the interviewer. Moreover, we feel it is important to be honest and up-front with your concerns. Deceiving your child about what you're doing makes it harder to develop trust, and ultimately you'll need that trust if you're going to be successful. Still, telling your child you're planning to seek professional help often leads to an uproar. Be prepared for your child to try to dissuade you from undertaking the consultation. Your child may object to missing school for the appointment or point out that you'll have to take time away from work, but you need to stand firm. The importance you place on this appointment sends a message that will be key to your continuing to be active in getting your child's problem under control. Certainly we have had parents "drag" their child in for an evaluation with us, but this is not the norm. Instead, a clear message that the pediatrician has made this referral, that you are concerned, and that this visit will help clarify the situation is usually enough to get the child to the expert's clinic. Then it's up to the experts to do their job in providing a helpful assessment and set of treatment recommendations.

Whom and What to Look for in an Evaluation

Actually, in our experience, the second problem—getting a good evaluation for an eating disorder in a child or adolescent—is in some ways the greater problem of the two you face once you've decided you need help. Many communities don't have resources to assist with diagnosing and treating children and adolescents with eating disorders, particularly professionals who are up to date on the best techniques and approaches. It is clear that we cannot solve this problem with this book, but we hope that from the outset, by emphasizing the seriousness of the problems that eating disorders cause, we can encourage parents to make an effort to seek out regional expertise in the area, even if it is not available at the community level. We liken eating disorders to any other serious medical problem—such as leukemia or heart disease—for which it is often necessary to travel a bit farther to specialty centers for consultation and initial evaluation and treatment to achieve the best outcomes. In the Resources section of this book, we provide a guide to regional centers of expertise that we hope will help parents locate experts closer to them. At the same time, the following paragraphs provide a description of our evaluation process to help you know what to anticipate when you do have an expert consultation, based on processes at our treatment centers.

Once a referral has been made and an appropriate expert has agreed to meet with the patient and parents, an evaluation will probably begin with the clinician meeting alone with the adolescent. This provides a developmentally appropriate entry into the family that respects the adolescent's developing autonomy. The adolescent should expect to be interviewed with support and warmth, with the clinician minimizing presumptions of understanding. Open-ended questions about family, schoolwork, interests, and activities are used to break the ice with reluctant adolescents. Open-ended questions also provide an opportunity for the adolescent, when willing, to offer his own perspective on what's happening to him and what's motivating him and to express whatever level of discomfort he experiences with eating. This open-ended approach is also important because not presuming an understanding of what's happening, but still being clear about what needs to be explored, is the most objective way to gather information in a clinical interview.

It's important, of course, that the interview focus on eating behaviors and problems, but most clinicians will find that they need to collect a significant amount of other relevant information. This other information includes such things as medical problems, other behavioral issues (with adolescents this includes drug and alcohol use), perspectives on other family members, and any history of traumas or abuse. The interview identifies any history of concern about weight and shape or health that preceded the onset of dieting or other behavioral efforts to change weight and shape. Adolescents will be asked about their exposure to common triggers for dieting and weight concerns, such as those mentioned earlier: hearing comments (positive or negative) on their weight, experiencing the onset of menses, dating, being involved in or exposed to family conflicts, starting middle school or high school, breaking up with a romantic partner, observing others beginning to diet at home or in their social circle, and so forth. The clinician should compile a detailed history about your child's efforts to lose weight. Examples of such behaviors include counting calories, restricting fat intake, fasting, skipping meals, restricting fluid intake, restricting meat and protein intake, increased or excessive exercising, binge eating, purging behaviors (exercise, use of laxatives or diuretics), and using stimulants and diet pills (over-the-counter items, health food products, and illegal products). Adolescents who binge eat and purge usually go through a cycle leading to increasing frequency of dieting, followed by binge eating and compensatory purgation. Persons with either anorexia or bulimia nervosa can binge eat and purge. However, those who are at extremely low weights because they are restricting their eating are more likely to call a much smaller quantity of food a "binge" than normal-weight adolescents who binge eat and purge.

Health consequences of these behaviors should also be evaluated. Adolescents with eating disorders commonly report chest pain, dizziness, headaches, fainting spells, weakness, poor concentration, stomach and abdominal pain, and cessation of menses. For those with bulimia nervosa, throat pain, involuntary regurgitation, broken blood vessels in the eye, and swollen neck glands are also common. Because eating disorders are often accompanied by anxiety disorders, depression, personality disorders, or obsessive–compulsive disorder, the interviewer will ask about symptoms of these disorders as well.

In addition to those areas specific to eating problems, interviews will include an evaluation of other possible contributors to the development of the disorder, including physical and sexual abuse, traumas, and emotional and physical loss. Some elements of this aspect of the interview will be necessarily private, and the contents will not be shared with you as parents unless warranted.

After the interview with the adolescent, you will usually be interviewed without your child present. If there are two of you, both of you need to be present. Your respective perspectives on your child and family are otherwise unavailable. You will be asked about the general development of your child—complications during pregnancy, early feeding, developmental milestones, transitions to preschool and elementary school, aspects of attachment (such as problems with separation when you dropped your child off at preschool, excessive clinging or irritable behavior when you were separated from your child, refusal to spend the night with friends because of fear of separation from you), early temperament and personality traits, family problems during childhood, and peer and sibling relationships. Your perspective on who your child is and how your child may have come to have this problem creates an atmosphere of shared understanding and often makes it easier for the clinician to proceed to the specific history of the eating and weight problems that have brought you to the practitioner's office.

Next you will be asked how you saw the problem developing: When did you first perceive a problem? What have you tried to do to help? Do you see other kinds of emotional or developmental problems, such as depression or anxiety, peer problems, or other changes in behavior in your child? It's likely that the evaluation will compare information obtained during the interview with the adolescent with the parents' version of events and will explore commonalities as well as differences. Together, these differing perspectives help generate a more comprehensive narrative of the events leading up to and sustaining the current eating problems.

> Charlotte agreed to meet with the psychiatrist reluctantly. She did not want to miss school, and she said she was eating well. In the interview, Charlotte said she had lost weight because her stomach was bothering her—she had had the flu a few weeks ago, and her stomach was still recovering. She denied having

any desire to lose weight and said she had eaten a muffin and juice for breakfast; a sandwich, chips, and cookies for lunch; and pasta with chicken and cheese sauce for dinner the day before. She said she exercised for only half an hour a day. She denied any lightheadedness, weakness, or headaches. She did admit to having skipped her menstrual period for the past 2 months.

When the clinician met with Charlotte's parents, they reported a very different version of events. Charlotte had begun losing weight about 5 months earlier. She did have the flu, but she had already lost 20 pounds by then and had lost another 5 pounds during that illness, which she had failed to gain back. Her parents reported that Charlotte had eaten about two bites of a muffin the morning before and drank about 4 ounces of juice. They also said they had regularly found Charlotte's lunches in the trash. Charlotte also exercised for at least an hour a day and hardly ever sat down anymore.

Sometimes clinicians who treat eating disorders ask for consultation from a dietitian with expertise in working with eating disorders. Sometimes dietitians calculate a target weight, which is derived from norms of weight for height in the patient's age group. Alternately, they may calculate the body mass index, defined as follows: weight in kilograms ÷ height in meters^2. Either way, these weights serve as a general guide to determine a reasonable weight range for recovery. This can be helpful in clarifying the degree of weight loss or weight gain your child has experienced and how far off he is from expected growth and weight norms for his age, maturity, and height. Dietitians can also provide educational advice to you, your teenager, and your doctors about the need for proper nutrition for health.

THE CHALLENGES OF DIAGNOSING AN EATING DISORDER

At the end of a proper consultation, if warranted, your child will likely receive a diagnosis of one of the major types of eating disorders. However, it is possible that the assessment will lead to a diagnosis of another problem that initially resembled, but is not, an eating disorder. Sometimes a fear of choking can lead to refusal to eat, and this may also look like anorexia. In this case, appropriate treatments would be for other conditions—depression and anxiety—rather than for an eating disorder.

Diagnoses are made to help clinicians decide on the best treatment recommendations for specific problems. So that you understand what the evaluating clinician means when rendering a diagnosis of your child, we think it is important that you know how eating disorders are described in DSM-5, the standard reference for diagnosing psychiatric problems in the United States, which was revised in 2022.

> Carlos had been overweight his entire life. Both his mother and his older sister were overweight as well. When Carlos started eighth grade, he decided he would go on a diet. His parents supported this idea, because they felt it would improve his health and self-esteem. Carlos was determined in his dieting and lost 10 pounds in a little more than 2 weeks by eating and drinking very little and beginning an exercise program of walking and jogging. Over the next 2 weeks, Carlos increased his exercise and continued to eat very little. He lost another 5 pounds. He became increasingly focused on his dieting. He got up early in the morning to go for a run and stayed up late doing "crunches" and leg lifts. Over the next month, Carlos lost another 5 pounds. He was now at a normal weight for his height, but his parents noticed that he was not satisfied. Carlos said he wanted to lose another 20 pounds. Teachers reported that Carlos was having trouble paying attention in class. Carlos said he was just going over the calories he had eaten during that day. He was still getting good grades, but he no longer had time for friends because of his exercise program. His parents tried to get Carlos to eat more, but he refused.
>
> When Carlos went to see a psychologist, he was told he had an eating disorder. Carlos protested that he wasn't too thin and he wasn't throwing up his food. The psychologist pointed out that Carlos was totally preoccupied with losing weight, food, counting calories, and excessive exercise. Carlos countered that he was just "getting healthy" and that he was tired of being fat. Carlos began to cry when told he needed help.

When reading about Carlos, it is not clear whether Carlos is in the early stages of anorexia, may be at risk for developing bulimia, or will develop binge-eating disorder. What is clear is that Carlos has an eating disorder and needs help.

Although you will be faced with the dilemma of how to get started, as we've described here, you should be less uncertain about when to act. Now is the time. The one thing you can be certain of is that once eating disorders become established, they do not give up their firm emotional and physical grip on your child. We know that for both anorexia and bulimia nervosa the longer someone has the illness, the more difficult it is to treat. For anorexia, for example, we have little evidence of any effective treatments after someone has been ill for several years. In the case of bulimia we know that a chronic course, in which symptoms come and go for periods of several years, is a common pattern when the illness goes untreated. A delay in taking action only facilitates increased habituation to these illnesses, making it harder for you to succeed in helping your child. So act now!

FOR MORE INFORMATION

American Psychiatric Association, *Diagnostic and Statistical Manual of Mental Disorders, Fifth Edition,* 2013. Washington, DC: American Psychiatric Association.

Brownell, K. D., and B. T. Walsh, Editors, *Eating Disorders and Obesity: A Comprehensive Handbook, Third Edition,* 2017. New York: Guilford Press.

Le Grange, D., and J. Lock, Editors, *Eating Disorders in Children and Adolescents: A Clinical Handbook,* 2011. New York: Guilford Press.

Lock, J., *The Oxford Handbook of Child and Adolescent Eating Disorders: Developmental Perspectives,* 2012. New York: Oxford University Press.

CHAPTER 2

Get Together

Everyone is confused.

Bridget refused to eat with her family. Her mother told her father that Bridget was going through a phase. She just needed time to make her own decisions. Bridget's father disagreed. He felt she was stonewalling the family and shouldn't be treated differently from anyone else. Bridget's sister was mad that she still had to eat dinner with her parents and little brother. Bridget's little brother said he missed Bridget and asked how come she didn't eat with them now.

No one knows what to do.

Bella has had anorexia nervosa for 2 years now. She meets with her therapist twice a week and her nutritionist once a week. Bella says her therapist tells her that she needs to decide to eat and get better and that her parents should stay out of it. The therapist said as much to her parents as well. The nutritionist advises Bella on what to eat and how much. Bella's parents aren't sure what Bella's weight is or what the nutritionist is recommending, but Bella remains very thin and her food choices are still quite limited.

You are frightened and angry.

For the third time this week, Sam is making a trip to the bathroom just after eating dinner. Sam's father follows him to the bathroom at a safe distance. Through the closed door Sam's father hears the shower being turned on, and a few minutes later he hears a coughing and choking sound. Sam's father stands outside the door and begins to cry silently.

You are helpless.

You've just left the pediatrician's office. Laila has gained another 5 pounds since her visit a month ago. You have found fast-food wrappers under her bed and in her closet. You hear her creeping down the stairs at night and wake up in the morning to see the wastebasket full of discarded cartons and packages.

You've given up.

Sam has just stormed away from the dinner table again. All you were asking was that he finish what was on his plate. This is a fight you've been having since he was 4 years old. Your husband says he was the same way at Sam's age, but the pediatrician says Sam is falling off his growth curve. But you're tired of fighting. Your husband will just have to figure it out without you.

You've been told by therapists and friends and you've read in books and online that if your child has an eating disorder you should stay out of it and let the therapist help your child work on the issue. You're told that this hands-off approach is the correct one because a salient feature of eating disorders is the need to control something. Adolescents with eating disorders reportedly feel "out of control," and it follows that this makes them feel anxious, so they seek to control the one thing they think they can control—what they eat. You also may have been told that these feelings of being out of control probably arise from things you did as a parent. You may have been told you were either too intrusive and overinvolved and controlling, or too distant, underinvolved, and abusive. Either way, it seems you could be the source of the problem, and therefore how can you be part of the solution? In fact, the farther away you are, the better.

You've heard all these things, but they don't feel right to you. How can you stand by and watch your daughter starve herself or listen outside the bathroom door while your son throws up his dinner? How do you explain to your other children that you know their brother or sister is not eating or is binge eating or is throwing up, but that you're trying to help by letting their sibling "manage" it alone? They don't buy it. Your other children are already trying to get your son to eat more and to quit throwing up. These things don't feel right to you because your gut sense as a parent is that it is somehow wrong to stand by and do nothing when one of your children is suffering. It also doesn't make sense to you because you know that you should be able to help. You *need* to help.

Why is it so hard to find a way to help with eating disorders? You would know what to do if your child had another kind of problem, even a very serious one like cancer—you'd take her to the hospital, get the best doctors, support your daughter during radiation therapy, surgery, or chemotherapy by being with the child. You would make sure that you understood the medicines, and you would make sure your child took them. You would make sure your daughter got to all scheduled appointments for follow-up visits, and you'd be on the lookout for signs of relapse or problems.

In other words, you would be a part of helping, no matter what. You would take off work or quit work if needed. You would borrow money to pay for treatment. You would question the doctors, and you would carefully evaluate all their recommendations. You would not leave all decisions up to your child, because you know that your child wouldn't or couldn't fully appreciate the repercussions of complicated decisions and options. You would do these things because you are a parent.

In contrast, when your child has an eating disorder, you are often left to your own devices. You don't know what's being done in terms of treatment. You're not sure about what options there are. You are told not to interfere with the therapist's and nutritionist's recommendations. You are told to butt out.

> After her third hospitalization in 5 months for a low heart rate and blood pressure due to starvation, Mandy's parents were fed

up. Each time 13-year-old Mandy came home she had promised to eat more. There were always excuses. Mandy's therapist felt she wasn't trying in therapy. Mandy's nutritionist said she wouldn't see her anymore unless she agreed to eat more and gained weight. Mandy's pediatrician felt she should be sent to a residential treatment center, where she would get 24-hour-a-day care, individual therapy, group therapy, dance therapy, pet therapy, recreational therapy, medications, and art therapy. Her parents would be 500 miles away. Mandy didn't want to be sent away. She was trying her best.

Seventeen-year-old Tony is throwing up every day at school after lunch. The boys hear him doing it and have told the guidance counselor. She has now called you. Tony says he's got the flu one day, ate something that didn't agree with him another, or just doesn't answer at all. He says he's quitting school if you send him to a shrink.

You wonder why eating disorders are so different from other illnesses. Why shouldn't you be able to help? Isn't there a way to help? There *must* be a way to help.

There *is* a way to help.

HOW THE NATURE OF EATING DISORDERS PITS PARENTS AGAINST THEIR CHILDREN

You know that your son has changed since developing an eating disorder. You've observed that your child is more distant, seems depressed or moody or irritable, and is obsessive about food (and probably other things). In some cases your child's already pronounced tendencies toward perfectionism are further accentuated. In other cases he's become more irritable, moody, and inflexible. Actually, your child's driven nature is more pronounced, period, whether in a good way or a bad way. What has happened?

We like to use a Venn diagram to describe what has happened (see Figure 2.1). One circle (white) represents your child before the eating disorder started. The other (black) represents the eating

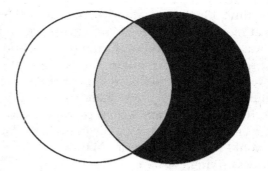

FIGURE 2.1. How an eating disorder overshadows your child's true self.

disorder. Over time, the eating disorder circle increasingly overlays the circle that represents your child. Her circle pattern is still there and recognizable but is now being altered by the eating disorder. So, many of her traits, though still present, are colored by the eating disorder. Say, for example, she tends to be perfectionistic. This trait is still present, but now it is particularly evident in connection with food—precise calorie counting, exact measuring, obsessive label reading, and so forth. Or perhaps she is anxious. Now her anxiety is increased at mealtime, and she refuses to eat around family or friends. Driven qualities can also be redirected. She now exercises for 3 or 4 hours a day at increasingly intense levels. We like to say that the eating disorder is using your child's characteristics (often great strengths but also sometimes weaknesses) against her. That's one of the reasons it's so hard for your child to battle the illness on her own—she's fighting herself and her own determination, drive, perfectionism, emotional lability, inflexibility, and obsessiveness. This combination of your child's characteristics and those of the eating disorder is confusing. You recognize your child's personality traits, and yet there are these major changes in focus—about food, weight, and exercise. This makes it difficult to know how to proceed. Some of the very things you may value in your child now stand in the way of your being able to help her. Here's an example: Your child is an exceptionally talented ballet dancer. She develops anorexia nervosa. You see her losing weight, but she gets a principal role in the dance school's production. Her talent, persistence, and ambition are paying off, but they are also being used to further the physical and emotional devastation of anorexia nervosa. As a parent you're torn between supporting your child's talent and allowing anorexia nervosa to become further entrenched.

Maybe that example is too easy. Suppose your daughter is a high school marathon runner. She is likely to be one of the best in the state. However, she has started throwing up and not eating so as to improve her performance. Her performance does improve. Still, she exercises more and more. Her performance begins to deteriorate. You know she has an eating disorder and should quit the team, but your daughter cries that without running she will get depressed and will kill herself. That's all she cares about.

Here's yet another example: Your child is preparing for the SAT. (In the United States, this is the Standardized Aptitude Test most young people take if they wish to go to college.) She's gotten straight As and is taking advanced placement courses. Her SAT scores, though, are not as high as they need to be to clinch her admission to the prestigious college she aspires to. In addition to having anorexia, she has become an overly dedicated student—staying up very late at night and getting up very early—in preparation for retaking the SAT, which is about 8 months away. You see that her focus on schoolwork is actually helping to prevent her from eating normally, and you hear her exercising late at night when she's taking a break. She tells you she has to study for the SAT and needs to exercise to keep awake. You want her to get into the college she wishes to attend, but you also see her becoming thinner, with darker circles under her eyes, and increasingly withdrawn from friends and family.

All the preceding examples demonstrate how the nature of eating disorders is confusing for parents and can pit them against their child. However, there are other ways that eating disorder symptoms lead to conflicts between parents and children. One of the most bedeviling problems is the timing of these illnesses. Anorexia nervosa, bulimia nervosa, and binge-eating disorder often occur just when adolescents are both more able to be independent and certainly very interested in being so. Thus, you are battling both the symptoms of the illness and the developmentally appropriate stage of increasing independence. In other words, sometimes you don't know if you're struggling with an eating disorder or with typical adolescent strivings for autonomy. When your child says to you, "I'm old enough to make my own decisions about what I eat," there is a ring of truth to it. The only problem is that often when adolescents make decisions because they have an eating disorder, and battle for them, the fight is "fixed"—the eating disorder wins, and both you and your child lose.

> Lidia had always been fiercely independent. When she was a preschooler, she spent hours learning to tie her shoes rather than let someone help her. Her parents had always respected Lidia's spirit and supported her when she struggled with the task, because they could understand what she was trying to accomplish on her own. As a young teenager, Lidia had chosen her own classes, decided who her friends would be, and chose her own clothes. Not surprisingly, when she began losing weight and her parents tried to step in to help her, Lidia was strident in her opposition. She fought over every morsel, filled herself up with water, and refused to eat anything her mother cooked for fear that her mother had put butter in it. At first her parents chalked this up to normal teenage rebellion and delayed taking any definitive action about treatment. Lidia continued to lose weight and then began binge eating and purging. Now they realized that the things they were fighting Lidia about were not normal teenage issues, nor were they rational problems. They were evidence that Lidia's thinking had gone awry and that an eating disorder had developed.

Along with this striving for independence, with adolescence comes increased wishes for privacy. This too helps eating disorders along. Eating disorders tend to increase secretive behaviors to avoid detection and thereby prevent intervention. So, because of others' respect for these adolescent needs for privacy, eating disorders can go on for months and even years without anyone really appreciating their presence. This is true despite the fact that adolescents themselves often leave abundant clues. Some save all the packages from the food they consume in boxes under their beds. Others vomit into plastic containers and save them in their closets. Still others lose a great deal of weight and hide under sweatshirts and baggy clothes.

Even if you've noticed some of these behaviors, it feels like prying to ask about them. Such is the power of an adolescent's need for privacy.

For children with avoidant/restrictive food intake disorder, common personality traits and behaviors are inattentiveness, anxiety, inflexibility, oppositionality, and hyperactivity. These are often exacerbated by undereating, low weight, and conflicts about when, what, and how much to eat. For many families the eating disorder and these traits and behaviors seem inseparable: Where does avoidant/restrictive food intake disorder end and your child begin?

It's pretty clear that the symptoms of eating disorders, your child's personality traits, and the expectations for autonomy and privacy during adolescence make it difficult to know how to take on this problem. How can you?

HOW CURRENT APPROACHES TO TREATMENT CAN REINFORCE CONFUSION ABOUT THE FAMILY'S ROLE

The main approaches to treating adolescents with eating disorders are family therapy, individual psychodynamic therapy, cognitive-behavioral therapy, and dialectical behavioral therapy. These approaches are important clinical interventions that undoubtedly help many adolescents with eating disorders. At the same time, some of the ways these approaches conceive of parental involvement can be problematic both for your child and for you as a parent.

There are long-standing debates about the role of parents in the treatment of eating disorders, particularly anorexia nervosa. The earliest physicians to describe the treatment of anorexia nervosa disagreed about this. In the late 19th century, Charles Lasègue in France felt parents were essential to treatment, whereas Sir William Gull, just across the English Channel, proposed that parents were the "worst attendants." Many current approaches either exclude or blame parents, explicitly or implicitly, causing parents to be confused about whether and how they can help their child with an eating disorder. In addition, because of the severity of both the psychiatric and medical problems of anorexia nervosa, hospitalization or residential care is often recommended. This requires separating the child with anorexia nervosa from you and other family members. "Parentectomy" is seen as desirable and is still common in Europe, though the costs of these types of long-term hospitalization have become very burdensome in the United States.

Short of a parentectomy, some individual approaches to the treatment of adolescents with eating disorders in the outpatient setting also advise strongly against parental involvement. These approaches view the young adolescent with anorexia nervosa as having an inadequate sense of self resulting from a problematic relationship with her parents, usually her mother. This inadequate sense of self is supposedly due to insufficient nurture and respect for the child's needs and failure to sufficiently separate maternal needs from those of the developing child. These developmental failures lead to the child's developing an identity based on overcompliance with parents' and other authorities' expectations, with little sense of her own needs and wishes. During adolescence this compliant strategy falters, but because of fear of parental rejection, feelings of powerlessness, and little sense of her real wishes, the teenager turns to extreme dieting and an irrational pursuit of thinness as a way of expressing her internal anxieties about separation and individuation. She feels "out of control" because she does not have the internal resources to cope with the independent thought and action required during adolescence and adulthood. A focus on what she can control, her weight and food intake, provides reassurance that she has some identity—albeit one devoted to the sole pursuit of thinness. In this way anorexia nervosa becomes intricately bound up with the developing sense of identity, making it difficult to challenge.

Certainly, many adolescents with anorexia nervosa do seem to struggle with the typical adolescent issues. Nonetheless, the implication that treatment should be focused only on the adolescent through her relationship with a therapist to "re-parent" her is questionable on several grounds. First, there is little scientific evidence supporting the notion that parents, and mothers in particular, of children with anorexia nervosa systematically differ from others in how they have parented their children. Most parents of children who develop anorexia nervosa have other kids who do not develop the disorder but were generally parented similarly. Studies of the feeding practices of mothers whose children later develop anorexia nervosa show that they don't appear to differ substantially from typical feeding practices. For example, although one researcher found that "picky eating and early introduction of solid foods" predicted more eating disorders in adolescence, the same practices when used with siblings did not lead to eating difficulties. Furthermore, studies of parental psychopathology as an indicator of overinvolvement with children don't provide clear evidence that these parents truly differ from others. The studies suggesting that this is the case evaluated families who were in crisis about their child's starving, making it impossible to draw conclusions about their functioning without this stress. In other words, even those studies that find evidence of intrusiveness and overinvolvement in families in which a child has an eating disorder can only say that these differences were present once an eating disorder had developed, but not before. This is important, because it is this presumption—that parents, in particular mothers, have *caused* the problem of anorexia nervosa in their children—that supports the clinical notion that they should be excluded from treatment.

> Jamal was always good at school, though he was somewhat shy. He didn't really like rough sports, but he excelled at tennis and swimming. When he developed anorexia nervosa at age 14, his parents took him to a psychiatrist who said he believed that Jamal was struggling with being independent and was confused emotionally and sexually. The psychiatrist suggested psychoanalysis as a way to help Jamal address these problems instead of avoiding them by starving himself. His parents wanted only the best for their son, and they had the resources to pay for intensive psychotherapy—anything to help him.
>
> Jamal was happy enough at first to go to therapy. He was never a disobedient child. Even as a teenager, he seldom mouthed off or complained about his parents' requests. However, over time Jamal complained about time away from his homework (he was in an honors class in all subjects) and from his workout schedule, which included a 2-hour swim in the morning and a run in the afternoon. He said he liked this therapist. They talked about his friends and his parents, but not much about eating or weight.

His parents dutifully took Jamal to therapy four afternoons a week. However, after a few months, they didn't see any improvement. In fact, they felt Jamal was getting worse. He was still losing weight and he was eating even less. His therapist had told them to let Jamal decide what to eat and when to exercise, and they deferred to this recommendation, though they were constantly worried. Things came to a head when Jamal began to refuse to go to therapy. He said that he didn't see any reason to go and that he was better. His parents could see that he wasn't.

Other adherents of individual therapy have excluded parents for developmental reasons. Developmental theorists have suggested that to support adolescent autonomy, parents should be, in the main, left out of treatment. To support age-appropriate autonomy, some clinicians contend that it is the adolescent herself who must take on the challenge of anorexia nervosa, more or less as a preamble to beginning to emerge as an adolescent once again. Parents, according to this school of thought, will simply reinforce the preadolescent stance, furthering anorexia nervosa's regressive hold on their child.

Gary was on his high school's rowing crew and had developed anorexia nervosa initially while trying to be as fit and as lean as possible to better succeed at this sport. When Gary's parents took him to a therapist, she suggested that Gary was struggling with a wish to be more independent but was frightened of the responsibilities of work and relationships that being more grown-up would entail. She suggested that Gary needed help with being more self-assertive and that he should be given more control over his life as was appropriate for a 16-year-old boy. Gary's parents agreed that he should be independent, but they thought that at this point he was too ill to make good decisions and were worried about the consequences to his health if he made poorer ones. Risk taking and exploration are a part of adolescence, the therapist explained, and it was necessary to trust Gary more and let him make mistakes if need be.

Gary competed avidly on crew and his team did well, but by midseason he was no longer able to participate because he had lost additional muscle mass and wasn't strong enough to row even short distances. Gary said he understood that he had made a mistake and would now eat more to gain his muscle back. He did this for a while but became anxious about getting out of shape and once again cut back on eating and increased his exercise. Gary's parents wanted to step in to help their son, but because they wished to respect his adolescent need for independence, they held back.

You only have to think about the behavior of children with anorexia nervosa to see that the illness effectively stops adolescent development. It throws children off the normal trajectory of physical maturation (ceasing menstruation, for example), encourages them to isolate themselves from the peers with whom they need to start to align to acquire independence, and leads to their being more involved with their parents and family, because of being ill, than would be usual for a teenager. But why would this necessarily lead to a conclusion that adolescents with anorexia nervosa should face the challenge of battling this illness without a great deal of parental involvement? After all, kids don't generally face the challenges of adolescence without parents. In fact, the presumption that having a stormy, conflict-ridden relationship with their parents is a necessary rite of passage for all teenagers no longer has much support. We now know that the teenagers who function best are those who continue to make productive use of their parents during adolescence—whose parents develop skills that enhance and support their adolescent children's progress through this stage of burgeoning autonomy. This may be even truer for adolescents who have difficulties of one kind or another. That is, teenagers who not only face the predictable challenges of adolescence but also have a physical or emotional problem are likely to need to rely even more on parental resources to ensure their ultimate success with and mastery of the tasks of adolescence. Thus, it may be all the more important for teenagers who develop anorexia nervosa to be able to garner the support of their parents in their struggles with the illness.

Many believe that the fundamental issues driving the development and maintenance of eating disorders should be addressed in individual therapy rather than through parental management. Eating disorders are often described as illnesses of "control," and so it is assumed that "taking control" away from the adolescent with regard to eating and dieting will exacerbate the problem. It's true that eating disorders lead to high levels of anxiety about food and weight, and indeed this anxiety decreases, relatively but briefly, when patients feel they are controlling these parts of their lives. Nonetheless, the anxiety returns rapidly and with renewed insistence, leading to even greater restriction and control, resulting in a cascade of increasing weight loss and worry. Patients report their mind-numbing preoccupations with counting calories, reading recipes, counting fat grams, weighing, measuring, special cookware, plates, and so on. The misery that accompanies these preoccupations is tolerable only because of the relief from the anxiety, which occurs intermittently, that reinforces these behaviors.

If, however, eating disorders are diseases of control, the sense of control is quite illusory. Patients do not feel in control; rather, they feel a *need* to feel in control. This difference is crucial. The pursuit of thinness, weight loss, dieting, and so forth is a search for control, not true evidence of control. In this sense, contending that the adolescent needs to remain in control of her eating and diet is a fabrication because when she has an eating disorder she does not have this control to begin with; instead, she is constantly trying to reassure herself that she will get such control. In this sense, the adolescent with an eating disorder is in need of someone to take control or at least help her take control, rather than leave her with an ever-shrinking ability to meet the behavioral and psychological demands of her illness.

Ironically, treatment modalities that advocate parentectomy to a greater or lesser extent, in the name of giving the adolescent control over food and weight, actually take most of the control away. Hospital programs regularly insist on consumption of set amounts of food or liquid supplements over which the patient exercises no control. Dietitians regularly prescribe dietary regimens for patients to follow. Some refeeding programs (professionally administered programs designed to rapidly restore weight) simply resort to nasogastric refeeding rather than involve the patient in even the activity of chewing and swallowing. Still, upon discharge, parents are told to let the child manage her food choices on her own. What is interesting, though, is that most younger patients experience a brief period of relief of anxiety when they are treated in such programs. That is, when someone else takes control of their eating and weight, they can often allow themselves to let go of the anxiety about these concerns. This accounts to no small degree for the success of these inpatient refeeding programs in treating the acute weight loss and malnutrition associated with anorexia nervosa. If most people with an eating disorder simply rejected these interventions, these programs would not succeed.

Why don't people with eating disorders rebel against these intrusive procedures as they do at home? It could be argued that it is against their nature to be confrontational and directly rebellious. Others report that these people have supreme (and somewhat justifiable) confidence that they can undo this weight gain rather quickly once they are allowed to be in charge again. Both of these perspectives are likely true, but certainly the latter point is not contested. Though most refeeding programs succeed in helping people with anorexia eat more in the hospital (or other intensive settings), many lose the weight gained and revert to their restrictive behaviors when left to their own devices upon discharge. The question then is how best to build on the progress accomplished in these programs.

> Lilly was a precocious 10-year-old who developed anorexia nervosa after she lost weight at summer camp. She was hospitalized for severe starvation. In the hospital, Lilly at first protested against eating and yelled and cried for her mother. She complained about missing her family and her friends. She hated missing school. Members of the nursing staff, who were quite experienced with these behaviors, provided a consistent presence at mealtimes and quietly insisted that Lilly eat her meals. They waited with her, encouraged her when needed, and set a limit on how long she had to complete her meals. Meals were provided at regular intervals, and snacks were also served routinely. Lilly gained weight and seemed less troubled by her eating symptoms, and after 3 weeks was discharged home.
>
> Lilly almost immediately began to restrict her eating again. Her parents were unsure what to do, although they now knew more about anorexia nervosa than they did before. Lilly said that she and the nutritionist had worked out a meal plan that she was supposed to follow. Her parents didn't really understand it. Meanwhile, Lilly started school immediately and threw herself

into the work with her usual vigor. As she studied more and once again became preoccupied with her grades, she ate even less. Within 2 months Lilly was back in the hospital, weighing even less than she had when she was first admitted.

Another reason parents have been excluded from individual treatment is the assumption that parents of children with eating disorders are unduly focused on weight and dieting. The theory is, somewhat reasonably, that parents are the vehicle through which children and adolescents learn about and filter their experiences of the culturally informed thin ideal. Parents who emphasize extreme concerns about weight in themselves, others, or their children are seen as likely to promote body dissatisfaction in their children, who internalize the thin ideal as communicated by their parents. For this reason, treatments focused on helping with body image dissatisfaction or, more important, body image distortion, exclude parents, who are seen as the likely suspects in causing this increased reliance on the thin ideal as a source of self-evaluation. Although it is undoubtedly true that parents can influence dieting concerns and behaviors, few support the distortions associated with eating disorders even if they have the illness themselves. Instead, parents can and often do serve as a reality check on these distortions and thereby likely mediate the influence of other social and cultural pressures, such as the use of alcohol and drugs, sexual activity, and social role performance.

Yet another reason that parents may be excluded from treatment is that many therapists believe that it is the parents who have caused the illness or are doing things to make it worse. Families themselves have been implicated in the etiology and maintenance of anorexia nervosa. The most famous formulation of the family as the cause of anorexia nervosa is based on the psychosomatic family process as observed by Salvador Minuchin and colleagues. These clinical investigators characterized psychosomatic families (including families with a child with anorexia nervosa) as enmeshed, overprotective, conflict avoidant, and rigid and said that each characteristic led to difficulties for the adolescent in negotiating the transition to adolescence:

1. In enmeshed families, the needs of the individual were unclear and difficult to assert.
2. Overprotective families prevented adolescents from engaging in the necessary social and psychological risk taking crucial for developing autonomy.
3. Families that tended to avoid conflict thwarted the necessary strivings for independent thinking and behavior.
4. Rigid families had difficulty adapting to the necessary change in role and function associated with having an adolescent whose needs were different from those of younger children.

In addition to these problems in family process, psychosomatic families were said to have structural problems, such as where children take up the role of a parental figure and/or where the parents, facing the developmental challenges of adolescence, abdicate responsibility. Other researchers have suggested that there may be problems in how parents are emotionally connected (attached) to their children with anorexia nervosa. Some feel these parents promote a kind of false independence by not relating sincerely and deeply to their children. If children develop this "false independence," it tends not to hold up during adolescence, and problems such as eating disorders may ensue.

> Lan and her family came to family therapy for anorexia nervosa after they had read that problems in families were often the reason children developed eating disorders. Lan's parents were professionals who had accomplished a lot in their respective careers. Her father was an accountant who traveled a great deal, and her mother was a physician. There were no other children. Lan had been a somewhat anxious child, but over time she had gained increasing confidence and had, to all appearances, sailed through elementary school both academically and socially. When she developed anorexia nervosa in eighth grade, it was the parents' first sign that there were problems.
>
> The family met with the therapist, who determined that Lan was too close to her parents, particularly her mother. Being too close to her mother interfered with Lan's need to be more independent as a teenager. In addition, and in part because Lan and

her mother were so close, Lan's father and mother, it was suggested, weren't acting together, and instead Lan was usurping her father's role. Finally, the therapist said, the family needed to address their suppressed anger. They needed to acknowledge their disagreements with one another. The family agreed to try.

For several weeks the therapist asked the family to describe their conflicts, which were at this point all about Lan's not eating. The therapist accepted that not eating was the subject of their arguments but suggested that not eating was just a symptom of other conflicts they weren't describing. The family was increasingly perplexed but tried hard to identify problems. Lan's parents spent more time together, as the therapist directed. Lan was encouraged to spend time outside the family, which she did, mostly by going on runs or going to the gym. Meanwhile, Lan continued to lose weight and had gone on to her eighth month without a menstrual period. Lan's parents asked the therapist when they could expect Lan to get better.

The research literature on the pathology of parents and families of adolescents with anorexia nervosa is fraught with difficulties, and conclusions are far from clear. Many researchers and clinicians argue that it is not the family that is causing some of the problematic behaviors seen in teens with anorexia nervosa, but rather the illness and the family's experiences of the illness. In other words, families become overprotective *because* their children are ill. They become enmeshed *because* they're trying to understand what's happening to their child and therefore appear intrusive and overinvolved. They want to avoid conflicts *because* they fear making things worse. They become more rigid *in reaction* to the stress the illness imposes on them. Although this debate is not resolved, the position taken by many clinicians is to presume the parents and family are guilty until proven innocent, thereby justifying the limitation of parental involvement in treatment.

Despite this stance by many clinicians, the notion that parents are unnecessary to treatment has been challenged increasingly over the years. Family therapists view the families of patients with anorexia nervosa as not only necessary to involve in treatment but essential to the recovery process. However, many still arrive at that conclusion because they see families as the "problem" in anorexia nervosa, and therefore neglecting to treat them would mean leaving the essential core of the illness to fester. It is only recently that parents and families of adolescents with anorexia nervosa have been perceived as being likely to exert a *positive influence* on bringing about recovery of anorexia nervosa but *not* being perceived as the likely cause of the problem to begin with.

HOW FAMILIES CAN COME TOGETHER TO FIGHT EATING DISORDERS

As we've said, many current therapies exclude parents and families, pay them only lip service, or blame them for causing or worsening the illness. However, family-based treatment (FBT) is a therapeutic approach that takes a different view. The basic tenets of this approach were first developed at the Maudsley Hospital in London in the 1980s and have subsequently been manualized, refined, and empirically tested. This form of family therapy doesn't blame the family but encourages its members to support their child actively by taking responsibility for helping their child eat normally, restore weight if malnourished, and normalize activity. This treatment, unlike many of the other currently used approaches, has been actually studied in a series of trials that provide evidence that it is helpful. Indeed, it's the only therapy for anorexia nervosa that has any substantive empirical support (see Chapter 6).

The basics of FBT are as follows. First, parents and the family as a whole are helped to understand how serious eating disorders are. To do this, the therapist reviews just how much the adolescent has changed, as well as the trajectory of serious problems (medical and psychological) that follow if the eating disorder goes unchecked. Next, the therapist helps family members see how important they are in changing the outcome, while reminding them of their abilities and previous successes in solving other family problems. The therapist also reminds parents that unless they are prepared to send their child away, it will be they who will have the ultimate responsibility for setting up an environment that supports improved behaviors related to eating and weight. This responsibility can feel overwhelming, and so parents are assured that the therapist will help them, not by telling them what to do, but rather by reviewing with them their successes and dilemmas and problem solving with them, using the resources that parents and siblings bring to help.

With this as an impetus, the therapist, using his expertise and experience, consults with parents in their efforts to change maladaptive eating behaviors. When working together with a therapist, most parents are able to make dramatic changes in such behaviors relatively quickly. When these behaviors have ceased to be the main concern, the therapist encourages the parents to help their adolescent manage eating independently, but with some guidance. Once the adolescent is managing eating and weight on her own, the therapist concludes treatment by strategizing with the family members about how they might address more general issues of adolescence. This helps prepare the family to leave therapy ready to proceed in the normal course of things.

We've been using this therapy in our centers for eating disorders in adolescents for over 25 years now. We have been involved in research, as well as in clinical work, using this approach that doesn't blame parents but helps them better help their children with the symptoms of eating disorders and provides ample opportunity for education and support. Consequently, we've seen adolescents with eating disorders improve dramatically. Not only do their symptoms abate, but, on the whole, the family also feels better able to negotiate adolescent issues in other areas. FBT has been adapted and shown to be effective for bulimia nervosa in adolescents and preliminary data suggest it is useful for avoidant/restrictive food intake disorder as well. In this sense FBT, or at least the main principles, is transdiagnostic—that is, applicable for all eating disorders in youth.

Even if this form of family therapy is not available to your child, adopting its principles, described in the following paragraphs, can help you find a way to be involved in your child's treatment, to the child's ultimate benefit.

1. **Parents bring important resources to their child's recovery and can be involved in whatever type of treatment the child receives.** It's the purpose of this book, in fact, to demonstrate how

Get Together

you can adopt this perspective to your child's benefit in a variety of clinical settings and treatment approaches.

2. **It's important for parents to take eating disorders seriously.** One insight that FBT highlights is the importance of realizing that eating disorders are serious medical and psychiatric illnesses. They are so serious, in fact, that as a parent you need to be highly aware of their potential for killing or severely damaging your child. Bulimia nervosa, anorexia nervosa, binge-eating disorder, and avoidant/restrictive food intake disorder are not just instances of taking dieting or problematic and disordered eating too far; they are truly *illnesses*. By emphasizing this principle, as we began to do in Chapter 1, we hope to help motivate you to take more immediate and definite action to help your child.

3. **You need to know what you're up against.** As a parent, you need to become sufficiently informed about the eating disorder so that you know how to evaluate to a reasonable degree whether your child is getting better or not doing well. Parents are prepared for many difficulties that their children may develop, but they are understandably not expected to know very much about eating disorders. Over the years it has become increasingly clear that parents' involvement is helpful in treatment for eating disorders in youth. FBT is now the approach recommended as first line for adolescents with anorexia nervosa and bulimia nervosa according to many national and international guidelines.

4. **It's not your fault.** The FBT approach includes a nonblaming attitude toward parents. If you feel guilty and responsible for causing the eating disorder, you likely also feel hopeless and inadequate when facing the task of trying to help your child change her eating behaviors. As we've said, though, we believe you are a key ingredient in your child's success in fighting the eating disorder. So it's our job, both in our practice and in this book, to alleviate any anxiety or guilt that is keeping you from contributing to your child's return to health.

5. **You need to be empowered to take up your parental role effectively.** Leveraging your love and abilities as parents in the

service of fighting an eating disorder is crucial. This is fairly easy to see in the case of anorexia nervosa, where the adolescent seldom has any motivation to recover. Without your strength, your child is left to the devices of the disorder and the downward spiral of weight loss and obsessional thoughts about food and calories. However, the same holds true for bulimia nervosa and binge-eating disorder, where the shame and guilt about the illness holds your son captive. For avoidant/restrictive food intake disorder, habit, unrealistic fears, and sensations of disgust often keep him from being able to change his eating behaviors on his own. When you are able to be a part of the process, these factors actually diminish as you support your child through these dilemmas.

6. **"Getting together" involves the whole family.** It's not just you who are a resource for your child. In fact, your whole family is able to help, in distinct but definite ways. Everyone in the family is affected when a child has an eating disorder. Everyone is worried or angry or both. Your other children see the effects on you and on their sibling. They are often most articulate about how much their brother or sister has been changed by the disorder or is affecting everyone else, especially at mealtimes. They also have clear memories of activities and qualities that are no longer present in their sibling with an eating disorder. Siblings can provide an avenue of support for their sister or brother who is ill, especially when your child may be angry at you for being firm about requirements for attending therapy or setting a limit on a behavior such as throwing up or not eating. They are also excellent sources of distraction and fun, which are needed when someone is fighting an eating disorder.

7. **The therapist is your consultant, not the boss.** In this sense, all therapy with children and adolescents must acknowledge the importance of family relationships. Therapists may be experts in particular areas, but they are not going home with you and do not routinely have to confront the problems in your home—they do not have to eat meals with your family regularly, clean up the bathrooms, and so on. That's what you do as parents. Therapists can help you think through problems and sometimes may even work independently with

your child, with your approval, support, and understanding, when needed. But, ultimately, you are the parent and they are advisers to you as you try to navigate the difficult problems that eating disorders present for you, your child, and your family.

So, there is a way you and your family can help your child who is suffering with an eating disorder. It involves, to start with, discarding the notion that you caused the problem. This idea is unproven and will cripple you in your efforts to help. Next, you need to learn all you can about how people with eating disorders think and behave, what motivates them to do what they do. When you do this, you are better prepared to counter them instead of being surprised and taken for a ride. Any therapist you find, regardless of her approach, should want to involve you. You should ask about how you will be involved and how you can help. According to some approaches, the therapist sees her job as helping you help your child, whereas other therapeutic approaches you may find attractive might see you in a more supporting role. In any case, you need to know what the treatment is, what its goals are, and what you will be doing to support it and your child. You should not sit back, but should instead take responsibility for your child. Don't let an eating disorder "de-skill" you as a parent; don't assume that you no longer know anything. Instead, assume you have a right to know what treatment your child is receiving, a right to look for ways you can help, and a responsibility to ensure that your child is getting the best treatment.

The rest of this book is designed to help you grow more confident in playing an active role in your child's (and your) struggle with an eating disorder. We hope to educate you more about what eating disorders are and how they can affect your child and family. We will review the kinds of treatment options you are likely to find and help you determine how you can be a part of each of these types of treatments. We also will provide you with examples of the kinds of problems you may face and how you might negotiate them. We hope this will help make you feel more empowered and, with that, even more capable and responsible as, with your help, your son or daughter combats an eating disorder.

FOR MORE INFORMATION

Bruch, H., *The Golden Cage: The Enigma of Anorexia Nervosa*, 1978. Cambridge, MA: Harvard University Press.

Crisp, A., *Anorexia Nervosa: Let Me Be*, 1995. Hove, UK: Erlbaum.

Le Grange, D., and J. Lock, *Treating Bulimia in Adolescents: A Family-Based Approach*, 2007. New York: Guilford Press.

Le Grange, D., J. Lock, K. Loeb, and D. Nicholls, An Academy for Eating Disorders Position Paper: The Role of the Family in Eating Disorders, *International Journal of Eating Disorders*, 2010, *43*, 1–5.

Lock, J., *Family-Based Treatment for Avoidant/Restrictive Food Intake Disorder*, 2022. New York: Routledge.

Lock, J., and D. Le Grange, *Treatment Manual for Anorexia Nervosa: A Family-Based Approach, Third Edition*, 2025. New York: Guilford Press.

Minuchin, S., B. Rosman, and I. Baker, *Psychosomatic Families: Anorexia Nervosa in Context*, 1978. Cambridge, MA: Harvard University Press.

CHAPTER 3

Don't Waste Time on "Why"

Is this my fault?

Stewart woke up at 3:00 in the morning again. His wife, Ariana, was already awake. They were worrying about their daughter Julie, who had anorexia. Stewart was lamenting the time he had spent talking to his children about the importance of regular exercise. Now Julie wouldn't stop exercising. Ariana blamed herself for focusing attention on good nutrition. Now Julie could tell you every food's calorie content and fat grams. Ariana was also berating herself for having fashion magazines at home. Now Julie spent an inordinate amount of time looking at herself in the mirror, pinching nonexistent fat on her stomach and thighs. Stewart and Ariana were sure they had somehow caused Julie's illness. They felt sick with guilt and overwhelmed with doubt about how to proceed.

Perhaps the biggest hurdle you face in trying to figure out how to help your child is the message, both covert and overt, that you must have caused this problem. Something you did as a parent, some failure on your part, some trauma you unconsciously inflicted on your child, resulted in the development of an eating disorder. As we'll discuss, however, the causes of eating disorders remain unknown, and your possible role is uncertain. There may be things we do as parents that increase the risk to our children of a variety of problems, both emotional and physical. However, none of those things we might do—for example, worrying about weight, being vegetarians, or eating unhealthily—appear to be specific enough to warrant being labeled a cause of eating disorders.

The truth is that causes of illnesses, especially psychological illnesses, are not easily discoverable. Remember, it took several thousand years to discover the bacterial and viral causes of illnesses like smallpox and pneumonia, and for infectious illnesses the line of causation is direct: Exposure to these bacteria or viruses will ultimately lead to the development of an infectious illness. (Although some attempts have been made to explain anorexia nervosa as a result of exposure to streptococcus, there is no evidence that this is the usual cause of this illness.) An explanation for how psychological illnesses arise, including those with a very clear genetic basis, relies on a much more complex theory of causation that is both indirect and interactive. It is fairly easy to show that by ridding the environment of certain bacteria, pneumonia won't develop. But it's impossible to rid the environment of genetics or vice versa (in fact, they evolve together and inform one another).

Despite the complexity involved in uncovering causation for psychological illnesses, and for eating disorders specifically, theorists have tended to support their recommendations for treatment on the basis of presumed causes. This is confusing and at times misleading. Psychological treatments clearly do not depend on specific knowledge of causation. If they did, we would have little hope of finding helpful interventions. This means that you don't need to understand what has caused your daughter's or son's eating disorder in order for them to recover. In fact, dwelling on what may have caused the problem often diverts parents' energies from helping their child. And like Stewart and Ariana, many parents who get mired in the question "Why" end up with nowhere to point the finger of blame but at themselves and then become paralyzed by guilt.

Although eating disorders have been around for a long time (some have cited evidence of eating disorders going back as far as ancient Egypt), modern recognition of these illnesses dates from the first descriptions of anorexia nervosa in the 1600s by Richard Morton and then in the late 19th century by Sir William Gull in England and Charles Lasègue in France. Since anorexia nervosa was first described, theories about the etiology of the disorder have ranged from viewing it as a purely physical disease to seeing it as the result of societal forces and not a disease at all. In contrast, bulimia nervosa is a much more recent phenomenon and was first described by Gerald Russell only in 1979 and was initially seen as "an ominous variant of anorexia nervosa." Bulimia nervosa as a distinct disorder has emerged over the ensuing years. Its cause is also unknown, but it is usually described as having biological, social, and psychological roots. Binge-eating disorder has been studied as a separate disorder from bulimia nervosa for about a decade but became a separate diagnosis only in 2013 with the publication of DSM-5. Avoidant/restrictive food intake disorder was included for the first time in DSM-5. The causes of these disorders are unknown.

A CLOSER LOOK AT INDIVIDUAL FACTORS IN CAUSATION

At this point in the evolution of our understanding, eating disorders overall appear to be multifactorial—that is, caused by the interaction of many factors. In the following pages we review some of the factors that theoretically contribute to causing anorexia nervosa, bulimia nervosa, binge-eating disorder, and avoidant/restrictive food intake disorder to help you understand (1) how little we actually know about the causes of eating disorders and (2) how assuming we know the cause can lead us down paths of treatment that may not be helpful.

Although it's certainly not a bad thing to have some theoretical ideas about the cause of an illness, when these ideas remain untested but still become gospel for therapists—as has happened for eating disorders, particularly anorexia nervosa—treatments that aren't based on these ideas often remain unexplored as well. And when these ideas center on parents' contribution to cause, they can remove parents as a key ingredient in recovery by disabling them through guilt and creating counterproductive therapist bias against them. The mental health field saw the same thing happen with schizophrenia and autism: The development of these severe psychiatric disorders was typically laid at the parents' doorstep until a deeper understanding of the biological causes of these illnesses was gained. By explaining what we do know about various potential causes for the eating disorders covered in this chapter, we hope to convince you that you are not to blame any more than parents of children with schizophrenia or autism are ever at fault. Putting self-blame behind you will restore your confidence in your ability to help with the problems that eating disorders present for your child. As you're reading about the *theorized* causes of eating disorders, remember that your goal is to go beyond these theories to embrace the need for change and begin to take action.

It's Biology!

Some interesting and important research is actually being done on the biological and genetic aspects of eating disorders. For example, studies show that anorexia nervosa and bulimia nervosa tend to aggregate in families, especially among first-degree female relatives. Eating disorders are three to five times more common in families in which a person is found to have such a disorder than in families in which no one has had an eating disorder. Still, of course, the vast majority of family members, male and female, do not have an eating disorder. One way researchers have tried to refine these observations about family clustering of eating disorders is by determining whether identical twins raised separately have similar rates of illness. Identical twins have exactly the same genetic makeup (or nearly so), so any differences in the occurrence of eating disorders between identical twins who are raised in different families are likely to be due to different environmental factors. Investigators have found that there's a significantly increased risk in twins that appears to be genetic rather than environmental. So, vulnerability to eating disorders appears to be inherited. Because, at least for now, we can't do much about our genes, we can't entirely blame parents, families, or society for the problem.

Not only do eating disorders appear to be heritable, but it's possible that certain personality traits and susceptibility to different behaviors may also be inherited. Traits such as perfectionism, obsessionality, anxiety, feeding behaviors, and negative mood states, which are associated with eating disorders, may also be heritable and thereby constitute particular vulnerability for developing eating problems. So far, researchers haven't figured out very much about this issue, but the idea is that eating disorders are caused indirectly, at least in part, by these inherited personality characteristics. It seems likely that this is true. The problem is that these characteristics may lead to very healthy outcomes. We've observed this many times. For instance, a young boy with anorexia nervosa has a mother who is a CEO and a father who is a doctor. They share many personality traits, such as perfectionism, drive, and obsessionality, but the outcomes are totally different, because in the parents these traits are applied to work, whereas in the boy they are focused on a preoccupation with dieting and weight.

Other research suggests that certain neurotransmitters are involved in vulnerability to developing eating disorders. Neurotransmitters are chemicals in the brain that affect a variety of brain functions, such as sleep, appetite, mood, and attention. When something goes awry with these chemicals, problems in any of these areas may result. Many neurotransmitters have been implicated in eating disorders (for example, dopamine, norepinephrine, and serotonin). Probably the most important neurotransmitters currently being studied are dopamine and serotonin. It appears that problems with regulating these brain chemicals are related to both anorexia and bulimia. Recent studies suggest that people with anorexia do not respond the same way to rewarding experiences (such as eating). Instead of experiencing pleasure, they are overwhelmed and anxious. It is suggested that being oversensitive to dopamine may be at the heart of this kind of anxious response. Studies using neuroimaging are trying to sort out these neurobiological aspects of eating disorders in more detail, and perhaps we will someday better understand the role of dopamine and other neurotransmitters in eating disorders.

For now, however, the exact nature of what goes wrong isn't clear, and, unfortunately, medications that aim to fix the problem (and that are effective for depression and anxiety problems) don't work as well with most eating disorders. They do, however, help somewhat with bulimia nervosa and binge-eating disorder. So, the argument goes that for some reason (inheritance, environmental stress, nutrition) something goes wrong with one or more of these neurotransmitters (or others not yet identified), which increases the likelihood that an eating disorder will start. Again, this may indeed be true, and medications may someday be of more help in treatment than they are now. However, focusing on neurotransmitters alone is unlikely to be enough because the attendant behaviors and thoughts appear to have a life of their own that is reinforced through habit and time. Unless those thought processes and behaviors are addressed directly, targeting neurotransmitters through medications isn't likely to "cure" the disorder.

> Dora was 13 when she began restricting her foods in an attempt to lower her weight. She had always been small and thin and did not like the idea of growing bigger. Dora was a bit of a loner. She could socialize with others when she had to, but she clearly preferred to read or study. She showed no romantic interest and shared none of her friends' enthusiasm for boy–girl parties. She was very close to her mother, who had seen Dora from an early age as a shy and vulnerable girl who needed her help to negotiate social challenges.

Gull and Lasègue's early descriptions of anorexia nervosa dovetailed with the emerging psychoanalytic movement in psychiatry and psychology that was to have profound influence on psychiatric treatment for half a century. Psychoanalysis is fundamentally a dyadic treatment (that is, one therapist meets with one patient). It also contends that psychological problems stem from early deprivations, traumas, and fantasies related to parents. The approach is basically designed to be used with adult patients (though Sigmund Freud occasionally treated children, and his daughter, Anna Freud, designed treatments for adolescents and children), whose fantasy life is explored through free association and dream interpretation. Patients with anorexia nervosa were seen as reasonable candidates for the psychoanalytic method, and their symptoms of self-starvation were interpreted in various ways. The early theoreticians relied heavily on Freud's understanding of sexual repression as the origin of all mental illness, and as a result, their theories of anorexia coincide with this idea. Thus, early psychoanalytic theory focused on guilt and oral impregnation fantasies, with weight loss seen as a defense mechanism—that is, "not eating" was a way of avoiding sexual thoughts and feelings. Although it has been observed that patients with anorexia are often sexually avoidant and may struggle with interpersonal intimacy, it's not clear whether this is more a result of the disease (starvation, for example, leads to lower sexual hormone levels, and this in turn leads to lowered sexual desire) than the cause.

Later, but still based in the psychoanalytic tradition, Hilde Bruch suggested that the person with anorexia is suffering from an "inadequate sense of self." By this she meant that the patient was socially immature and psychologically underdeveloped. As a result of not feeling confident and assertive, such adolescents turn to other ways of expressing their feelings, especially their anger. Thus, restrictive eating and related disturbed eating patterns are seen as forms of "acting out" the frustration and feelings of inadequacy that these adolescents experience. To assist with these problems, psychoanalytic treatment aims at helping to "find a voice" for this deficient self that substitutes psychological understanding and expression as opposed to disturbed eating as a way of communicating. Indeed, these adolescents often seem immature, naive, and not particularly assertive as compared with their peers. In fact, the theoretical idea that adolescents with anorexia nervosa need help with finding a sense of identity makes a great deal of sense. How to help them best accomplish that task in the context of a serious illness such as anorexia is less clear, but some approaches such as adolescent-focused therapy (AFT) in adolescents and enhanced cognitive-behavioral therapy (CBT-E) in adults appear to be effective.

Other recent research has suggested that some of the problems people with eating disorders may have could be related to *how* they think. Studies suggest that adults with eating disorders show problems in being flexible in their thinking style, which makes it difficult for them to consider alternatives and to use therapy. We see this in the rigid rule-bound behavior in anorexia nervosa and in some cases of avoidant/restrictive food intake disorder, particularly in those with autism spectrum disorder. Other studies have found that people with eating disorders struggle with not seeing the forest for the trees and get lost in too much detail. An overfocus on details makes it easier to perseverate and obsess rather than see the consequences of ongoing problems. We can see this with anorexia nervosa and sometimes with bulimia nervosa and binge-eating disorder when a person cannot appreciate the medical and psychological impacts of their disorders. Still, it remains unclear just how these problems in "thinking style" may relate to the risk for developing an eating disorder, whether in some cases they are simply a result of the disorder, and whether they can be addressed in treatment. All of this is under study.

It's All in the Family!

> Hiro's parents did not get along. His father was a busy surgeon, and his mother participated in many charity events and social activities. They seldom had overt conflicts, but they also were seldom together. Hiro's father left for work at 4:30 in the morning and returned after dinner. Hiro's mother was often out in the evening at fundraising planning meetings. When Hiro stopped eating, no one noticed for quite some time. By the time his father finally asked Hiro if he was losing weight and arranged for a physical exam, he had lost almost 25 pounds. When the family sat down together for therapy, it was the first time they could remember having been together for several weeks.
>
> Heather's mother had sent her to live with her father when she was 12 because she and Heather were fighting all the time. This arrangement went all right until Heather's father remarried. Heather and her stepmother did not get along well. Heather felt picked on, and her stepmother felt she wasn't respected. Heather moved back with her mother. During this period, Heather began to diet and throw up. She said she felt fat and ugly and no one liked her. She had few friends and was very isolated. Her mother was also quite busy with her own work and social life.

When family therapy arrived on the scene in the 1960s and 1970s, it was—as we noted earlier in this chapter—developed from a psychoanalytic base. Like practitioners of psychoanalysis, many family therapists see anorexia nervosa as a symptom of underlying pathology, this time located in the family as a whole. Therefore, conventional family intervention tries to modify perceived problems within the family or, if this fails, to remove the child from the family. Yet another form of family therapy, so-called structural family therapy for anorexia (probably the best-known approach), was devised based on clinical observations of families by Salvador Minuchin (a pioneer in family therapy for anorexia nervosa). Because the child played a critical role in the family's overall avoidance of conflict, self-starvation was seen as powerfully supported by the family, though its members were not aware of this. Structural family therapy tries to alter family organization by identifying and challenging what are believed to be inappropriate alliances between parents and children, encouraging the development of stronger sibling support of one another, and promoting open communication. The aim is to reduce the child's emotional involvement with parents and to improve the effectiveness of the parents. So this approach also strongly supported the idea that families, and particularly parents, are in some way the cause of anorexia nervosa and without help will only perpetuate the problem. Data on the idea that families of patients are truly "pathological" are surprisingly conflicting. Some studies suggest that these families do have unique problems of the type that Minuchin described, whereas others don't appear to detect differences between these families and so-called normal families. Even if there are such differences, though, it isn't clear how they relate to the development of an eating disorder. In other words, a family can have many problems (as in Heather's case), but the direct link between such problems and their causing an eating disorder is a *leap* that cannot and really should not be made.

It's a Stage. She'll Outgrow It!

Mimi has always been a good student but "slow to warm" socially. When her family moved to another city at the beginning of her sixth grade, it was not very surprising that she struggled to make new friends. She complained about the new school and about being lonely. She fantasized about going back to her old town, where she was happier and felt more accepted. Just after the winter holiday, Mimi had her first menstrual period. She told her mother that it hurt and she didn't like it. Although her mother tried to be supportive, Mimi remained very upset. Not long afterward, Mimi began to diet. She told her mother that she had an upset stomach or was too nervous to eat. Over time she ate less and less, and her parents became increasingly concerned. When the gym teacher called to ask Mimi's parents to meet with her about Mimi's weight, they were not surprised, but they didn't know what to do, either.

Eating disorders generally begin during adolescence. It is principally for this reason that many theorists have viewed the disorders as related to issues of this developmental period, specifically with struggles for autonomy. A model for the cause of anorexia was developed by Arthur Crisp, a London psychiatrist, who speculated in the 1970s and 1980s that anorexia was the result of phobic avoidance of adolescence. That is, Crisp suggested that adolescents who developed anorexia were anxious about the physical changes associated with puberty, about establishing a more socially independent identity, and about entering social relations as sexually mature beings. The weight loss that resulted from excessive dieting and exercise restored the body shape and hormonal status of preadolescence, and the medical and psychological secondary effects returned the adolescent to the more dependent status of a younger child. Therefore, the child apparently accomplished her goal of avoiding adolescent struggles. This theory, which is said to apply to adolescents with an eating disorder, shows a healthy respect for the normal processes of adolescents and families and provides a very good context for thinking about therapy for teenagers. Still, it is unclear how best to employ the insight that developmental issues are key to understanding eating disorders. Moreover, in a certain sense the theory raises the question of causation: After all, the developmental challenges associated with adolescence are common to everyone, so why do only some teenagers develop eating disorders in response? No one knows for sure. However, AFT—to be discussed in a later chapter—is one approach designed to address these developmental and interpersonal concerns without implying blame or causation, and instead focus on maintaining beliefs, cognitions, and behaviors.

It's Hollywood!

> Darnell spent hours studying himself in the mirror. He compared himself with the male models and athletes he saw in magazines. He felt his arms were too flabby and undefined. He wanted to be "cut" and lean. He wanted a "six-pack" of abdominal muscles. He began with lifting weights and cutting down on desserts and fast foods, but soon he was counting calories and throwing up to make sure he would lose weight. His friends noticed that he was looking very muscular and trim. Several girls talked to him and flirted. Darnell was sure he was on the right track.

Yet another approach to determining the cause of eating disorders focuses on the social and cultural forces impacting developing adolescents that may lead to increased problems with eating behaviors, body image concerns, and poor self-esteem. Although these forces have been influencing adolescent girls for some time, it's now clear that the same forces are acting on boys more than they used to. Several forces are considered likely culprits: notably, media images, Western cultural ideals, and wealth. However, because shape and weight concerns are not part of avoidant/restrictive food intake disorder diagnostic criteria, these social forces are not likely risks for developing this disorder.

Media

The forces imposed by the media influence children at a fairly early age. For girls, Barbie dolls and similar toys set very early standards for unrealistic expectations with regard to body shape and size. For boys, male images of unrealistic body mass and musculature are increasing as well. When the Han Solo action figure based on the *Star Wars* movies first came out in the 1970s, he had human proportions, but the more recent action figure is unrealistically muscled. In addition, studies of *Playboy* and *Playgirl* centerfolds document a continuing trend toward ever-decreasing body fat and greater leanness in the male and female models represented. Even a cursory look at a fashion magazine or television program yields a host of examples of very thin women and men with extremely lean and muscular bodies modeling the latest styles. The basic difficulty is that these toys, images, and models set an unhealthy standard for beauty that vulnerable children and young adolescent males and females then aspire to.

> Lia wanted to be a model when she grew up. She bought all the fashion magazines she could find. She shopped at every opportunity and spent a lot of time getting dressed for school and outings. During her second year of high school, Lia went to a modeling agency. She was told that she had a good face, but she needed to lose 15 pounds if she wanted to be considered. Lia was not overweight, but she decided that becoming a model would be worth losing those pounds. Lia began dieting, exercising, and taking diet pills to curb her appetite and laxatives to "cleanse" her system. She lost about 8 pounds, and her friends and family said she looked great. However, Lia felt she could be thinner. She continued to restrict her intake, but when she did eat, even a normal meal, she would throw it up.

Western Cultural Ideals of Beauty

That the popular media have a great influence on all our lives, especially the lives of adolescents, is obvious. Social values surrounding food and weight have long influenced our behavior. In the 16th century, for example, being overweight was "in," which made eating in abundance desirable, whereas being unduly thin was a mark of social inferiority and even sickness. In the Pacific islands of Tonga, eating disorders were unknown and overeating and corpulence were considered desirable until television was introduced in the early 1990s, after which eating disorders started to appear and young girls and women began to worry about their weight and to diet.

Western ideas of beauty and body shape are permeating other cultures all over the world, particularly in Asia. In the past several years, eating disorders have apparently been developing rapidly in Japan, Taiwan, Singapore, and Hong Kong. Studies of immigrants suggest that young women who move from a non-Western culture to a Western culture are at increased risk for eating disturbances.

> Indira's parents, both engineers, moved to the United States from India when Indira was about 2 years old. She had done very well in school, excelling in both academics and athletics. However, at the beginning of high school, Indira began to lose weight and to complain about her skin color. She asked her parents for blue-tinted contact lenses. Indira explained her desire to lose weight and wear blue contact lenses as a way to fit in better with her mostly White friends in the private school she attended. Her parents were concerned about Indira's developing identity and saw her anorexia nervosa as a manifestation of her conflicts about being a minority person in a White majority group.

Indira's description of her experience is in line with some cross-cultural studies suggesting that immigrants, especially non-White immigrants, are experiencing increasing problems with eating disorders. Among these adolescents there seems to be an increased cultural strain, that is, an increased need to "fit in" and be "acceptable" relative to the White cultural thin ideal. To accomplish this, some teenagers try to change their appearance, particularly their weight, to become more desirable and to compete more successfully. Becoming psychologically and emotionally invested in meeting Western standards of beauty regarding thinness causes some of these young people to pursue unhealthy weight-loss strategies to the point where they develop eating disorders.

Related to the problems inherent in the Western idea of beauty are feminist perspectives on eating disorders and their development. The basic idea is that Western ideas of beauty, in their focus on thin body ideals, are part of a large cultural attack on women and women's bodies that is designed to keep women disempowered. This is accomplished by setting unrealistic standards of attractiveness. When women feel they don't meet these standards, the result is low self-esteem, poor self-worth, and less ability to perform in the culture. In addition, of course, these feelings and perceptions lead to eating disorders—an effect of this larger attack on women.

The feminist perspective on the development of eating disorders is instructive in several ways. First, it integrates the ideas of beauty, power, and gender, which are common themes in patients with eating disorders. It also synthesizes the roles of culture and media in the development of eating problems. Furthermore, it suggests that even women in the wealthier classes (see the next section) are not immune. Although not usually articulated, the feminist perspective also provides a partial rationale for why and how eating disorders might be more common among gay men. However, it has less to say about eating disorders among heterosexual men, athletes, and religious persons, who are less likely to be victims of media and other mainstream social forces identified in the feminist literature in the same way.

Over the past decade, with the growth of social media and its ever-increasing use by youth, it has become evident that communication of the value of thinness, fitness, and beauty is even more prevalent and propagated by social influencers and artificial intelligence (AI) algorithms. In addition, AI tools to modify body and facial features add to the distortion of body parts and increase body shame.

Wealth

Eating disorders, especially anorexia nervosa, have long been associated with higher socioeconomic status. The maxim "You can never be too rich or too thin" captures the essence of this association. There are several possible origins of this relationship. The first is rather concrete: The wealthy no longer have to worry about basic survival, and being thin manifests this freedom. The second is more subtle: That is, wealth confers a special status—a superior status—such that one doesn't need to eat. Of course, the confluence of wealth and fashion fuels the fantasy that to be rich is to be thin and vice versa. In fact, it appears that anorexia nervosa may cluster more commonly among wealthier families, but it remains an equal opportunity disorder and can and does occur among all socioeconomic classes, ethnicities, genders, and racial groups.

However, it is less clear that wealth itself is the risk factor. It may be that some families are wealthier in part, as we have suggested earlier, because of some temperamental or personality traits that when applied to business lead to work and success, but when applied to dieting lead to anorexia. Thus, it may be a tautology to see wealth per se as the cause of anorexia. On the other hand, other eating disorders such as bulimia and binge-eating disorder don't appear to cluster to the same extent according to socioeconomic status. Instead, they are more widely distributed socioeconomically, culturally, and racially. Yet it may be that patients with bulimia are more sensitive to the influences of culture, media, or status (wealth), and this sensitivity may contribute to the development or maintenance of their eating-disordered behaviors, but how much or how specifically is speculative.

It's Due to Trauma!

There is a long-standing association between mental illness in general and sexual abuse and trauma. Researchers have been particularly interested in sexual abuse and eating disorders because many young women with eating disorders reported experiences of this kind to their doctors or therapists. Some studies have found that sexual or physical abuse is, in fact, a risk factor for eating problems, particularly bulimia nervosa, but no specific link between eating disorders and abuse has been established. The basic theory is that sexual trauma may heighten anxieties about the body, exacerbating an already exaggerated emphasis on weight and shape and leading to the development of eating-disordered thoughts and behaviors. Although certainly reasonable, this theory is not applicable to everyone, inasmuch as most people with eating disorders have not been abused or traumatized. And just as with targeting neurotransmitters, focusing solely on abuse or trauma seems unlikely to alleviate eating disorder symptoms, which take on a "life of their own" over time and need to be addressed specifically. The dilemma for therapists seems to be that it's easy to make sexual abuse or other trauma the sole focus of treatment because abuse is such a devastating event. Yet doing so, in our opinion, might make it more difficult to treat the eating disorder.

The role of trauma in the etiology of some children and adolescents with avoidant/restrictive food intake disorder appears to be important. Many report that the precipitant event to avoiding food was a choking incident. After this kind of event, some children become worried that they will choke and perhaps die and they are therefore afraid to eat. However, for those with persistent lack of interest in eating or who are just very picky, trauma appears to have little if any role. Instead, biological and personality factors are more likely to increase risk for avoidant/restrictive food intake disorder.

DON'T GET STUCK ON "WHY"

If it now seems that all the reasons proposed for developing an eating disorder make sense—or that none of them do—rest assured that both of these statements are true. It's a matter of perspective. It is also true that focusing on why your child has developed an eating disorder may not be very helpful. Imagine your child does not have an eating disorder, but cancer. No one knows exactly why she developed cancer, and the treatment prescribed does not aim at the cause of the cancer but instead targets the effects—removal of the malignancy and treatment with radiation and chemotherapy to prevent the growth of new cancerous lesions. Treatment for many childhood cancers is remarkably effective, even though the cause is often unknown and the treatment doesn't necessarily aim for it. For many of the diseases we treat in medicine, this is also the case. With diabetes, for example, we often don't really know why the body stops making adequate insulin, but we can control the disease with medications. Another example includes some types of seizures. We can generally identify the part of the brain in which the electrical impulses have gone awry, and sometimes we can perform surgery to resect that part. Usually, however, more conservatively but just as effectively, we treat the disorder with medications and the seizures are controlled. The list could go on. The point is that for most illnesses we have to treat symptoms—and in many cases we end up doing away with the disease in the process—but for mental illnesses we expect treatment to focus on eradicating the cause. This is largely because psychological and psychiatric research has been so interested in psychological explanations and conflicts, and this applies particularly to eating disorders. As we've seen, though, we seldom *know* what the cause is. How can we hope to eradicate the illness if we treat it by trying to eliminate what we can only guess is the cause?

It's understandable for you to want to know why your child has developed an eating disorder. It seems a random and unfair event, causing worry, hazard, and difficulty for your child and family. It's also understandable that psychologists and psychiatrists find investigating cause fascinating. Unfortunately, although research into why eating disorders occur may eventually help us prevent them from developing, we think focusing on causation often lures clinicians and families off course. Dwelling on cause in treatment keeps therapists and parents from dedicating their efforts to the problem at hand—keeping the starving teenager before them alive and restoring her to health. With your child starving or throwing up in front of you, a discussion of her genetic vulnerability for anxiety and eating problems, how controlling you were as parents, how immature she is psychologically, and the problems of society's standards for beauty will likely be distracting and probably take you off track, at least initially. This is time you may not be able to afford to waste. In fact, such meditations and preoccupations sometimes play directly into the hands of the eating disorder by allowing the behaviors and thoughts to persist without confrontation and redirection, for longer periods and with more success. (More on this phenomenon is presented in Chapter 5.) We know that the longer a person loses weight, maintains low weight, purges, and binges (in other words, the more chronically ill she is), the less likely we will be successful in getting rid of the eating disorder. This is true for any illness. The longer you have diabetes before you are treated, the more difficult it is to control and the more problematic are the long-term effects. The same is true for cancer, heart disease, and other debilitating illnesses. That being the case, it's important to take action quickly and decisively rather than just ponder why.

Setting aside the question of "Why" may be easier said than done. We would prefer that the question be deferred or bracketed while the disordered eating behaviors and related health and weight problems remain unresolved. We see these problems as leading to a kind of thinking that is similar to trying to do therapy with someone who is inebriated: You just can't do it because that person can't process what you're saying. You've got to wait until she is sober, or at least somewhat sober, before you can hope to communicate with her. In the meantime, you have to get her sober. That means getting the alcohol out of her system and trying to keep her from drinking again. With eating disorders, at least at the beginning, we believe you have to do the same thing. Stop the behaviors that are leading to the problem and keep them from recurring long enough that discussions about the problems associated with the disorder can be approached.

Perhaps the most important reason not to get stuck on "Why" is that your child needs your help now. By your setting the problem of "Why" to the side, we hope that you will feel less ashamed and guilty, see yourself as an excellent candidate to help your child get the treatment and support your child needs, and involve yourself in that treatment with confidence and commitment.

FOR MORE INFORMATION

Anderson-Fye, E. P., and A. E. Becker, Sociocultural Aspects of Eating Disorders, in J. K. Thompson, Editor, *Handbook of Eating Disorders and Obesity*, 2004. Hoboken, NJ: Wiley, pp. 565–589.

Bulik, C. M., Genetic and Biological Risk Factors, in J. K. Thompson, Editor, *Handbook of Eating Disorders and Obesity*, 2004. Hoboken, NJ: Wiley, pp. 3–16.

Crisp, A. H., *Anorexia Nervosa: Let Me Be,* 1980. London: Academic Press.

Field, A., Risk Factors for Eating Disorders: An Evaluation of the Evidence, in J. K. Thompson, Editor, *Handbook of Eating Disorders and Obesity*, 2004. Hoboken, NJ: Wiley, pp. 17–32.

Kaye, W., J. Fudge, and M. Paulus, New Insights into Symptoms and Neurocircuit Function in Anorexia Nervosa, *Nature Reviews Neuroscience*, 2009, *10,* 573–584.

Klump, K. L., S. A. Burt, A. Spanos, et al., Age Differences in Genetic and Environmental Influences on Weight and Shape Concerns, *International Journal of Eating Disorders*, 2010, *43,* 679–688.

Klump, K., and K. Gobrogge, A Review and Primer of Molecular Genetic Studies of Anorexia Nervosa, *International Journal of Eating Disorders*, 2005, *37*(Suppl.), S43–S48.

Levine, M., and K. Harrison, Media's Role in the Perpetuation and Prevention of Negative Body Image and Disordered Eating, in J. K. Thompson, Editor, *Handbook of Eating Disorders and Obesity*, 2004. Hoboken, NJ: Wiley, pp. 695–717.

Morton, R., *Phthisiologia: Or, a Treatise of Consumptions*, 1694. London: Smith and Walford.

Nasser, M., *Culture and Weight Consciousness*, 1997. London: Routledge.

Nasser, M., M. Katzman, and R. Gordon, Editors, *Eating Disorders and Cultures in Transition*, 2001. New York: Brunner-Routledge.

Wonderlich, S., R. Crosby, J. Mitchell, et al., Eating Disturbance and Sexual Trauma in Childhood and Adulthood, *International Journal of Eating Disorders*, 2001, *30*, 401–412.

PART II

UNDERSTANDING EATING DISORDERS

CHAPTER 4

Know What You're Dealing With

The Complexity of Eating Disorders

We probably don't have to tell you that you can't solve a problem unless you know what you're dealing with. Every day, at home and at work, you take steps to figure out what you're up against before devising a strategy for attacking a particular challenge. Whether it's getting the car to run or your checkbook to balance, getting your assistant to be more productive or your sales force to exceed last year's gross, you decide on a solution based on your understanding of the problem. Helping your child overcome an eating disorder is no different.

As you now know, having read Part I of this book, eating disorders are enigmatic and idiosyncratic. There are lots of gaps in our scientific understanding of anorexia, bulimia, and binge-eating disorder. What we do know sets eating disorders apart from other psychiatric problems affecting children and adolescents, which has made treating them an ongoing challenge. The gaps in our understanding of these disorders stem from the fact that there is a comparative dearth of research on eating disorders in children and adolescents. To heighten our challenge in the treatment of eating disorders, myths and misconceptions about these disorders abound in the popular media.

It's essential that you know what you're dealing with if you're to help a child who has an eating disorder. In this chapter we give you up-to-date, scientifically based information on these disorders. With this foundation, your quest to help your child will gain the greatest possible chance for success.

We can't state this too often: Know the facts. It could save your child's life.

EATING DISORDERS ARE PSYCHOLOGICAL ILLNESSES WITH SERIOUS MEDICAL CONSEQUENCES

Talk about complicated: No other psychological illnesses affecting children and adolescents involve pathological thoughts, behaviors, and emotions that lead to such serious short- and long-term medical complications. Because these disturbances in the way individuals think, feel, and act, in turn, bring about a dramatic change in food consumption, eating disorders can cause physical illness perhaps more than any other mental illness currently known. This means that parents and health care providers must not only understand the psychological workings of these disorders and apply psychological treatments, but also be alert to what's happening to the child's physical health. In fact, it is fair to say that in most cases you should deal first and foremost with your child's medical status. Starvation poses several medical risks, as we elaborate on in the following pages. Moreover, many of the psychological symptoms you may have noted in your child are the direct consequence of these medical problems. Therefore, it is of paramount importance that your child enter a treatment regimen, whether outpatient, inpatient, or residential, that will attend to her medical status and provide a supportive environment in which the psychological workings of her disorder can begin to be explored.

How Are Eating Disorders Defined?

Eating disorders, as we explained in Chapter 1, are of four main types: anorexia nervosa, bulimia nervosa, binge-eating disorder,

Know What You're Dealing With

and avoidant/restrictive food intake disorder. There are differences between them, but they also share many features. We have to consider both the similarities and the differences when we ask the question "What is an eating disorder?" It's sometimes difficult to know at the outset which of the four eating disorder diagnoses will be the most accurate because over time as many as one-third to one-half of patients can eventually be diagnosed with two or more of the different types of eating disorders. Although we mentioned the specific challenges of making an accurate diagnosis of an eating disorder in children and adolescents in Chapter 1, it's important to revisit these issues, with an emphasis on helping you identify the overlapping as well as distinguishing characteristics of a particular disorder type.

> Annette, now 16, has been ill with an eating disorder since she was 12 years old. She has spent most of the past 4 years in and out of the hospital. As a result, it has been very hard for her to spend significant periods of time at home with her parents and siblings, to make and keep friends at school, and to have an opportunity to build and learn from meaningful relationships outside her family. In addition, she has fallen seriously behind in her schoolwork even though the hospital unit to which she is usually admitted provides schooling for the adolescents in its program.
>
> Every time Annette is admitted, she is severely emaciated, which requires her doctors to put her on strict bed rest with frequent visits by the nursing and medical staff. Eventually, her weight begins to approach healthy levels again and she is prepared to be discharged to her parents' care. At this time, however, her parents are always told to "back off" as Annette should now take care of her own eating. Unfortunately, every time she tries to eat on her own, she promptly runs to the bathroom to induce vomiting because she "cannot stand" feeling so "full."
>
> The nurses in the hospital would have prevented Annette from vomiting, but at home, following the doctor's advice, her parents are backing off. Consequently, Annette's weight, time and again, spirals downward as she checks in every week with her outpatient pediatrician. Her pediatrician is concerned about the speed with which Annette always manages to lose weight once she is discharged, and he is also very worried because her daily vomiting after every meal has caused her electrolyte levels

to drop well within dangerous levels. Every couple of weeks, Annette gets herself admitted to a medical ward to restore her electrolytes to normal levels. Although this is a life-saving necessity, it again takes Annette away from her home environment, her friends, and school. This cycle—going to an eating disorder inpatient unit, back home, and then in and out of the medical unit—as well as receiving a multitude of different medications, has been a sad routine for Annette and her family for many years now.

While the exact criteria for anorexia nervosa have varied with each iteration of DSM, the disorder is characterized by a mismatch between energy intake and physical needs that leads to significantly low body weight. Exactly how low body weight needs to be and how it is calculated have varied as well, but for adolescents this weight needs to account for age, development, sex, and height. In addition, this low weight and insufficient intake is associated with fear that eating will lead to weight gain and becoming fat. In younger children this fear may not be verbally expressed but associated instead with behaviors that suggest fear (avoidance, overexercise, slow consumption of meals). There is also a misperception of current body shape—believing that they are overweight or fat even though malnourished, an extreme emphasis on the importance of weight and thinness as a measure of self-worth, and, in younger children especially, a failure to recognize that malnourishment is a serious medical problem.

There are two subtypes of anorexia nervosa, a restricting type and a binge eating–purging type. In DSM-5, amenorrhea (loss of regular periods) is no longer required to meet diagnostic criteria. The level of severity (mild to extreme) in adults is based on current body mass index (BMI); in children and adolescents, severity is based on age and gender norms according to BMI percentiles. A BMI below the 10th percentile is considered to be consistent with the degree of malnutrition associated with anorexia nervosa. Alternatively, if longitudinal growth charts are available, deviations from individual growth trajectories can be observed.

In terms of the subtypes, some people with anorexia nervosa use only extreme dieting techniques by limiting their intake (called the *restricting subtype*), and others engage in binge eating and purging (use of vomiting, laxatives, other purgatives) behaviors (called the *binge–purge subtype*). But among the diagnostic criteria for anorexia, there is the suggestion that failure to grow, an event specific to childhood and adolescence, will substitute for meeting the usual weight-loss criteria.

Bulimia nervosa is also defined as having both behavioral and psychological components. Behavioral components include intermittent severe dieting strategies that lead to weight fluctuations while the person maintains an overall weight within the normal range. The disorder is characterized by repeated episodes of overeating (a binge-eating episode). These episodes must be discrete and time limited (an hour or two) and be associated with a feeling of being out of control or being unable to stop eating. In response to these episodes, behaviors to prevent weight gain that would result from overeating are undertaken (for example, vomiting, laxatives, diuretics, fasting, compensatory overexercise). These binge-eating episodes and compensatory behaviors are repetitive and persistent (for example, about once a week for a few months). Self-worth is highly related to body shape, size, and weight, and the disorder is not associated with anorexia nervosa.

The severity of bulimia nervosa (mild to extreme) is based on the frequency of compensatory behaviors. In addition, for someone to be diagnosed with bulimia nervosa, these behaviors should be accompanied by extreme beliefs and attitudes that overemphasize control of shape and weight as the sole or major way to maintain self-worth and self-esteem. Children and adolescents developing bulimia may not necessarily meet the frequency criteria (the number of binges and purges per week), as the illness is not so well established yet.

Binge-eating disorder is similar to bulimia nervosa except there are no compensatory behaviors. The binge-eating episodes are usually rapid, sometimes occur even when not hungry, are associated with being overfull, and are a source of shame, guilt, depression, or embarrassment.

In younger patients with binge-eating disorder, these criteria are sometimes hard to apply because binge eating may occur only when parents are absent, so the frequency may be lower. In addition, because children and adolescents often don't buy the food available to them, the ability to binge eat depends in part on food being in the home. For these reasons, some have argued that if your child reports feeling out of control when eating, this is a strong indication that a problem with binge eating is developing.

As noted in the introduction, another new diagnosis was added in DSM-5, called avoidant/restrictive food intake disorder (ARFID). Little is known about this disorder, but the key features include an ongoing failure to meet nutritional needs as a result of disinterest in eating; disgust at the taste, smell, texture, or look of specific foods; or an irrational fear that an unwanted physical response (for example, vomiting, choking, allergic reaction) will occur. To distinguish the disorder from anorexia nervosa and bulimia nervosa, there must not be body image worries or fears of weight gain. Importantly, these behaviors are not fully explained as resulting from other medical or psychiatric problems (for example, cancer, allergies). These behaviors lead to poor physical health, including malnutrition, poor growth, pubertal delays, enteral feedings, and vitamin or mineral deficiencies. These eating difficulties must also lead to psychosocial problems (poor school attendance, family disruptions, inability to socialize).

This disorder is associated with disturbances in psychological development and functioning. Some patients are very picky eaters who also display a particular fear of different or new foods. They are sometimes excessively sensitive to food texture, appearance, and taste. For the patients with a swallowing or choking event or fear that contributes to food avoidance, a specific event can sometimes be identified as having caused that fear. The ARFID diagnosis is also used for children who simply have a lack of interest in eating or who have low appetite. For many reasons ARFID can be confused with anorexia, but the main differences are that, unlike adolescents with anorexia, these children are not afraid of weight gain, have no shape and weight concerns, and make no efforts to lose weight. In fact, children are usually aware that they are underweight and may say they wish they could eat more and gain weight but are afraid to actually eat enough to do so.

Medical Complications of Anorexia Nervosa

In Chapter 2 we exhorted you to view yourselves as part of the solution to your child's eating disorder—advice that's difficult to take when your son or daughter is treating you as if you're crazy at best, an enemy at worst. In truth, living with a child who has developed anorexia can make you feel as if you *are* insane. The illness is publicly quite visible—the fact that your child is emaciated is plain for all to see (if she hasn't shrouded herself in baggy clothing to hide the skeletal frame that you have been pointing to), yet she very likely will insist that nothing is wrong. This view of an illness as nonproblematic or "perfectly normal" makes anorexia a disorder that we call *egosyntonic*. The adolescent with anorexia nervosa may very well view her illness with a sense of pride or achievement and protect the illness through denial. As a consequence, your child may not willingly seek or accept treatment. In fact, this peculiar characteristic of anorexia tends to make your job as a parent more difficult overall when it comes to the medical complications of the illness. Adolescents without anorexia nervosa may notice a particular physical ailment, such as stomach pain or a headache, and be more than likely to bring that knowledge or awareness to their parents' attention. In contrast, adolescents with anorexia nervosa will almost certainly not appreciate the potential seriousness of any of their symptoms and, consequently, will not bring up the issue with you, their parents. Likewise, if you should note anything that worries you about your adolescent's health, you will experience the uphill and frustrating battle of trying to convince your adolescent that something serious might be wrong and that there is a need to check with your family pediatrician.

> Let's say that you're Linda's mother. Linda is 17 and has always been slender. You weren't particularly concerned about this; after all, she appears to be happy, does well at school, and seems to get along with her friends. All the women in your family have been "slow starters" in regard to the onset of menses, and you haven't been very concerned about the fact that Linda has never had a period at age 17. Your concerns were also brushed aside a year ago when you took Linda for a visit with her pediatrician and the doctor said not to worry and put Linda on the birth

control pill. The reasoning behind the doctor's intervention was that the medication would start her periods and thus "take care of things." In the past year, though, you have noticed that Linda has become increasingly withdrawn, even looking depressed at times. She remains picky about her food and doesn't eat as much as you think she should, and you've begun to wonder whether her frequent running could be making things worse. You decide to ignore your pediatrician's words of comfort and take Linda to see someone who specializes in eating disorders.

After you, your spouse, and Linda have talked to a team of specialists, you all learn that Linda's health has been compromised to a much greater extent than anyone has imagined. It turns out that she meets the criteria for anorexia. In addition to your worries about her mood and the fact that she's much more isolated socially and not as confident as you thought your 17-year-old would be, Linda's physical symptoms have alarmed the specialty team greatly. The medical examination revealed that in addition to Linda's low weight, which has persisted for several years now, she suffers from osteoporosis (a condition of brittle bones that fracture easily, which is quite common in postmenopausal females but very uncommon in someone who is healthy and of Linda's age). Making things worse, it turns out that Linda is no longer 67 inches tall as her medical records have always confirmed. Now she has lost a full inch in height (losing height is, again, quite common in older females who suffer from osteoporosis, but highly unusual in someone as young as Linda). You learn from the psychiatric team that treatment for Linda is going to be very complex, for it will not only address her weight loss, which is something she dreads, but will also help her with mood and social isolation. At the same time, the medical part of the treatment team will have to address the lack of menses (being maintained artificially by the birth control pill) and figure out how best to make sure that further loss in bone density can be prevented.

There's no denying that all these health problems are disturbing, especially when the child herself is denying there's anything wrong. Parents can get so caught up in the battle over eating, however, that some miss the early signs that life-threatening starvation has begun. Once the adolescent has reached an obvious state of emaciation,

Know What You're Dealing With

one of the first telling signs that starvation has reached serious proportions is the loss of menstruation, in postmenarcheal girls and women, as body fat declines. What can be confusing is that, for some, amenorrhea sets in after relatively little weight loss, but for others, only very low weight triggers the loss of periods. As noted earlier, this may be especially true for adolescents who do not have firmly established menstrual cycles. For many reasons, it also becomes a confusing issue in the case of boys with an eating disorder, as there is no clear equivalent to loss of menses. If you're worried about a son who may have an eating disorder, you'll have to be alert to the signs of other medical complications, such as low heart rate, low energy, and low testosterone levels.

In addition to causing loss of menses, severe malnutrition usually leads to a variety of serious medical consequences. Several systems are impacted by self-starvation: the central nervous system and the cardiovascular, renal, hematologic, gastrointestinal, metabolic, and endocrine systems. The most significant acute problems are bradycardia, hypothermia, and dehydration. All these complications can become life-threatening. The most important chronic medical problems for adolescents with anorexia are the potential for significant growth retardation (your adolescent with anorexia may not maximize her growth spurt and may consequently fail to achieve optimal height); pubertal delay or interruption, which can have serious consequences in terms of menses and fertility; and peak bone mass reduction, which can lead to osteoporosis or osteopenia (an increased porosity of the bone associated with frequent fractures). In addition, many other side effects of malnutrition are often noted:

1. **Hypothermia:** Lower than normal body temperature. You may notice that your adolescent wears extra layers of clothing to try to stay warm even when it is warm outside.

2. **Hypotension:** Decreased blood pressure (a systolic blood pressure of less than 90 millimeters of mercury for adults). Low blood pressure generally has no clinical symptoms, so you might not notice that anything is amiss with your child. However, if it is associated with decreased tissue perfusion (for example, poor circulation

causing cold hands and feet, or slow healing of cuts), your child may have increased heart rate, sweating, lightheadedness, and pallor. This is called *shock*, and it is deadly.

3. **Bradycardia:** Decreased heart rate (for adults, fewer than 60 beats per minute) or a slow pulse. In someone with anorexia, this correlates with the severity of the illness but can be detected only by taking a pulse or performing an electrocardiogram.

4. **Changes in skin and hair texture:** Skin becomes dry and flaky, and hair becomes brittle and can thin out quite dramatically. This is perhaps one of the few consequences of starvation that you, as a parent, may begin to notice.

5. **Lanugo:** There is often a development of fine, downy body hair, most noticeable on your adolescent's face and the back of her neck. This is another way in which the body is attempting to accommodate to the slowdown in metabolism, essentially trying to maintain core body temperature. As with the other skin and hair changes, you might actually notice this growth of fine hair on your child's face or neck.

6. **Growth hormone changes:** There is often an increase in growth hormone secretion, which can be detected only through laboratory tests.

7. **Hypothalamic hypogonadism:** This describes a decrease in sex hormones, which causes an absence of menses and leads to infertility. Blood tests can reveal this condition.

8. **Bone marrow hypoplasia:** Decreased blood cell production, including a low count of red blood cells, white blood cells, and platelets, which leads to anemia. The anemia may contribute to your noticing your child being a bit more fatigued than usual. The lowered white cell counts have not been found to be associated with decreased immune functioning in the case of anorexia.

9. **Structural abnormalities of the brain, generalized atrophy of the brain, and occasional regional atrophy:** This describes a decreased size of the brain or parts of the brain. There are no clear clinical signs of this happening in your child; it can be detected only if you specifically request a neuropsychological evaluation.

10. **Additional changes in electrical brain activity:** The electroencephalograms (which show brain activity with electrodes placed on the head) of children with anorexia are often abnormal. You will not be able to see these abnormalities just by looking at your child.

11. **Cardiac dysfunction:** This may include peripheral edema, decreased cardiac diameter, narrowed left ventricular wall, decreased response to exercise demand, pericardial effusion, and superior mesenteric artery syndrome. Your adolescent may describe fatigue, decreased ability to exert himself, and a swelling of his legs. Cardiac complications are often lethal and can be confirmed only with the help of an electrocardiogram.

12. **Gastrointestinal difficulties:** Delayed gastric emptying, gastric dilatation, or decreased intestinal lipase and lactase, for example, may manifest itself in your child as abdominal discomfort; your child may complain about a sense of stomach fullness after eating very little. Again, only sophisticated tests will help you confirm the true nature of your child's gastrointestinal problems.

Although these complications are most typical for adolescents with anorexia, restricting subtype, several other complications that are related to binge eating and purging behaviors in particular should also be considered. These complications will be clearer once we've discussed the medical issues associated with bulimia nervosa.

Medical Complications of Bulimia Nervosa

>Nora, now 17, had been binge eating and purging since she was 15 years old. Over the past several months, as she neared her graduation, she felt increasing pressure to excel in school. Unfortunately, she was also being pressured by her boyfriend to become sexually intimate, something she was afraid to do because she was ashamed of her "thunder thighs" and her "fat stomach." She began to purge more frequently, resulting in blood appearing in her vomitus. She was increasingly dizzy when she stood up, and her heart would race. One afternoon, as she went to her car from school, she fainted. Her friends called 911,

and she was taken to the emergency room, where she was found to be dehydrated and anemic; she also had a low potassium level.

Bulimia nervosa is a more secretive illness than anorexia, making it easier for your adolescent to hide her symptoms. The medical complications are also not as evident as might be the case with anorexia, for most adolescents with bulimia usually have a healthy appearance. In contrast to anorexia, bulimia nervosa is described as *ego-alien*, which implies that the sufferer is embarrassed or ashamed about her symptoms and is therefore hesitant to seek treatment.

Children and teenagers with bulimia nervosa rarely approach the low weights associated with anorexia. In fact, although some patients with bulimia nervosa are quite underweight and others quite overweight, most fall within normal weight limits. Unfortunately, we don't have much research data on teenagers with bulimia. We do, however, know that doctors who see such cases find the same signs and symptoms that are typical of adults with bulimia. We can then assume that the medical complications of bulimia nervosa will be about the same for your teenage daughter or son as for adult patients. We don't have any mortality figures for bulimia nervosa in either adults or teenagers, but certainly the medical complications that sometimes require hospitalization—hypokalemia, esophageal tears, gastric disturbances, dehydration, and orthostatic blood pressure changes—can result in death. There are indeed case examples of adults with bulimia nervosa who died because of esophageal tears, with extensive internal bleeding. Because many teenagers with bulimia nervosa have periods of starvation similar to those of teenagers with anorexia, many medical complications of bulimia are the same as those of anorexia. However, because bulimia nervosa is mostly characterized by binge-eating and purging episodes, there are some unique medical complications that are more common in bulimia. These are as follows:

1. **Hypokalemic alkalosis or acidosis:** Low potassium level (less than 3.5 milliequivalents per liter in adults) and acid/base imbalance go hand in hand, because changes in the acid/base balance affect the functional potassium levels. With low potassium, you may

notice general weakness and malaise in your child. The most catastrophic effect of a low potassium level, however, may be abnormal electrical conduction in the heart, which can lead to death.

2. **Hypochloremia:** This condition describes low serum chloride levels resulting from the body's attempt to retain electroneutrality in the presence of an acid/base imbalance. The lack of chloride increases serum bicarbonate levels, which then leads to metabolic alkalosis. What this means is that the body has accumulated too much of an alkaline substance (for example, bicarbonate) and does not have enough acid to effectively neutralize the effects of the alkali. This can be detected only with blood tests.

3. **Dehydration:** Because of decreased body fluid, your child may have dry skin and complain of fatigue or lightheadedness upon standing.

4. **Renal problems:** These can include prerenal azotemia—acute and chronic renal failure. *Azotemia* describes increased nitrogenous wastes in the blood (urea and creatinine), which are a sign of kidney dysfunction. Azotemia may be associated with generalized fatigue, paleness, anorexia (loss of appetite), and swelling. *Prerenal* indicates that the cause for this condition is not within but before the kidney, such as reduced fluid volume associated with the dehydration of eating disorders. *Acute and chronic renal failure* describes kidney malfunction or failure.

5. **Seizures:** Seizures are abnormal, sudden, excessive discharges of brain neurons. During a generalized seizure, the type of seizure generally relevant here, your child may experience a loss of consciousness, muscle jerking, tongue biting, and urinary incontinence.

6. **Cardiac arrhythmias:** These are irregular heartbeats. Many adolescents with arrhythmias don't have any clinical signs or symptoms, although some might notice palpitations (most commonly), shortness of breath, chest pain, lightheadedness, and loss of consciousness. Arrhythmias can be lethal.

7. **Myocardial toxicity caused by emetine** (using ipecac syrup to purge): Cardiac muscle poisoning by ipecac may cause

cardiomyopathy, which may manifest itself in your child as loss of consciousness, fatigue, and arrhythmia. It too can be lethal.

8. **Enamel loss and multiple caries:** As a result of the tooth damage often caused by bulimia, your child may report frequent toothaches, or you may notice that the general status of her dental health (and appearance) has deteriorated. In cases of frequent vomiting over time, some patients have lost almost all their teeth.

9. **Swollen parotid glands, elevated serum amylase levels, and gastric distention:** Your child with swollen parotid glands may look as if she has "chipmunk cheeks."

10. **Cramps and tetany:** Tetany describes intermittent paroxysmal muscle spasms. Tetany may also be associated with nervousness, numbness, and tingling of the arms and legs.

A vital aspect in the care of patients with eating disorders is an appreciation for the medical complications of such illnesses. It is often too easy for both parents and clinicians to underestimate the severity of these illnesses. It is only when a comprehensive evaluation of the adolescent's medical status has been completed and medical follow-up has been established that the psychiatrist or psychologist can focus on appropriate treatment to address the eating disorder symptoms and the concomitant psychosocial issues. So, always make 100% sure that your child has received a thorough medical workup by a pediatrician who understands eating disorders. In addition, make sure you're present for much of this examination so that you can add information the physician will need to reach a complete understanding of your child's medical status. Too often we find that the illness, whether it's anorexia nervosa, bulimia nervosa, binge-eating disorder, or ARFID, prevents the young person from sharing all the vital facts with the doctor.

Medical Complications of Binge-Eating Disorder

The main medical risks associated with binge-eating disorder are those related to the development of obesity as a result of chronic binge eating. Obesity is a severe health problem for the United States as well as many other countries because it leads to diabetes, hypertension, ischemic heart disease, stroke, and probably mortality.

Medical Complications of ARFID

For youth with disinterest in eating, low appetite, and fear of adverse events (for example, choking, vomiting, allergic reactions), the medical risks are similar to those associated with malnutrition found in the list presented earlier for anorexia nervosa. These children can become severely underweight, require tube feeding, and sometimes require placement of nasogastric tubes or jejunostomy feeding tubes. In addition, they can suffer from pubertal delay, short stature, and osteopenia/osteoporosis. For those with extreme picky eating, many of the medical complications associated with obesity are also found in binge-eating disorder. Other nutritional deficiencies related to poor intake can occur—vitamin D deficiency, vitamin C deficiency (risk of scurvy), and others—leading to poor growth and increased risk of infections.

EATING DISORDERS ARE OFTEN ACCOMPANIED BY OTHER PSYCHOLOGICAL ILLNESSES

It's not uncommon for eating disorders to be accompanied by other types of mental illness, at least in adults. We have less information in this area regarding teenagers, but you should be aware of this possibility. Other disorders that occur at the same time as the eating disorder—a condition referred to as *comorbidity*—can complicate your child's treatment and possibly reduce the success of treatment if the comorbid illness(es) isn't (aren't) managed well.

> Maria was first brought in for treatment when she was only 12 years old. She was away on vacation with her parents for a few months prior to her first treatment visit. It was during this family trip that her parents noticed she was looking very frail, and they became concerned about her increasing "fussiness" over eating and her insistence on exercising at least once every day. At the

time Maria's parents first brought her in for treatment, there were also some early signs that this prepubertal young girl was a very determined, hardworking, fastidious, and even overly organized person. In addition to providing support and understanding toward members of the family, given the crisis they were all facing, one of the first goals of treatment was to guide the parents in helping Maria get her weight back on track. Without this weight gain, Maria would not have a fair chance of entering her anticipated growth spurt as she approached menarche. Moreover, without weight recovery (and continued weight gain, given that she was only 12 and needed to gain weight throughout adolescence), her body wouldn't be healthy enough to receive the trigger that would start her first period.

Although weight gain was proceeding well, it became evident that there was another difficulty at hand that might seriously complicate the family's ability to remain focused (for now) on the job of getting Maria's physiological and psychological development back on track. Maria was becoming increasingly ritualistic in almost all her behaviors. What this meant in terms of her day-to-day life was that the mere act of walking to school became an ordeal, for she couldn't step on cracks in the sidewalk. At school, she could look only at some kids but not at others. At home, she had to arrange and rearrange her room several times a day to get it "just right." Most of these rituals, together with the repeated thought that "I must think 'good' things," kept her from any weight gain, or at least Maria was convinced this was true.

Of course, all these activities made a routine day very hard for everyone in the family and left Maria very little time to enjoy being with her parents and siblings, visiting with friends, or doing any homework. At this point, understanding these thoughts and rituals better so that appropriate treatment could be started had to be added to an already stressful treatment regimen of weight restoration and medical follow-up.

Several more assessments were added to everyone's busy schedule, including more visits to the pediatrician and even a neurologist. A brain scan was completed to make sure that nothing was overlooked in trying to make sense of the increasingly debilitating obsessive–compulsive symptoms. Different combinations of powerful drugs, with potentially serious side effects, were started, all in the attempt to help Maria gain some control over the intrusive thoughts and tiring rituals. All in all, her treatment became very complicated, and Maria, her parents, and even the treatment team had trouble managing all the different components.

Obsessive–compulsive disorder, as in Maria's case, seems to be a common occurrence with eating disorders, especially anorexia, in just over one-third of patients with chronic anorexia, according to one report. Because addressing these debilitating symptoms involves a great deal of extra attention from the treatment team, such as additional interventions—cognitive-behavioral therapy, and often several medications—it is easy to see how the focus could be diverted from Maria's self-starvation. The challenge here is to address the comorbid illness but not lose track of the primary job: taking care of the eating disorder.

Depression is another psychiatric illness that's quite likely to occur in combination with a child's eating disorder. According to one study, as many as 63% of all patients with eating disorders have a lifetime history of depression. It's important, however, to determine whether the co-occurring depression is a primary (independent) diagnosis or the result (side effect) of self-starvation—a question best sorted out by your teen's psychiatrist or psychologist. Although it will not always be easy for your child's doctor to distinguish between these two forms of mood disturbance, effective treatment of your adolescent will depend on a careful and accurate evaluation of her mood.

Clinical depression and low mood because of an eating disorder are two different things, even though they may look very similar to you. If your child, in addition to her eating disorder, suffers from clinical depression, the depression may respond to medication, or it may persist even when the eating disorder has responded to treatment. Keep in mind, though, that many adolescents with eating disorders appear dysphoric and demoralized. This form of "depression" may certainly be the result of the eating disorder, inasmuch as poor mood is a frequent side effect of starvation. The same is true when your child engages in binge eating and purging: She could very well feel "blue," guilty, disgusted, demoralized, sad, and so forth because of these symptoms.

For clinical depression, you should make sure your child's psychiatrist considers psychotherapy specifically for the depression, and in some instances psychotherapy plus an antidepressant, as the primary treatment. If you and your child's doctor are convinced that her low mood is secondary to her eating disorder symptoms, you should monitor her mood closely to be sure it also improves as her eating disorder gets better. If that doesn't happen, additional treatment for the depressed mood might be in order.

Some researchers in this field argue that, in addition to obsessive–compulsive disorder and depression, there is a higher than expected comorbidity between **personality traits** and eating disorders. For instance, avoidant traits (characterizing someone who is overcautious when it comes to interpersonal relationships, who finds it extremely difficult to make friends and is very shy, and so on) and anorexia often co-occur, and a significant number of individuals with bulimia have borderline personality traits (they are very impulsive in their behaviors and have changeable moods, as well as great instability in relationships). Although this may be the case for adults with eating disorders, it's unclear whether personality traits *and* an eating disorder are applicable to adolescents or children.

Nonetheless, many researchers from a number of theoretical backgrounds have reported differences in personality makeup among teens with various eating disorders. What many of them show is that girls with anorexia nervosa are often very anxious, inhibited, and regimented, whereas adolescents with bulimia nervosa can be all of these, but some also tend to be more emotionally volatile, impulsive, and/or uninhibited.

You should, however, keep two things in mind when trying to get an idea of how likely it is that your child—or any child—has other psychological problems along with an eating disorder. First, we'd be oversimplifying the eating disorders if we were to see each disorder as clearly demarcated by eating disorder symptoms alone because both anxiety and depressive states often accompany these symptoms. Second, it is also possible that current studies overestimate comorbid illness among individuals with an eating disorder. It may be that many patients with eating disorders who are included in research projects come from specialized eating disorder clinics, and therefore the more seriously compromised individuals may be overrepresented among those studied. In reality, children and adolescents with eating disorders are quite varied, and although many of them have comorbid illnesses, many do not. For you as a parent, the important point is to be aware of the possibility and alert to signs that something else may need the attention of your child's mental health care team.

Finally, **alcohol and drug abuse** are also commonly diagnosed in adults with bulimia nervosa, though no studies have documented this in younger patients. Many teens, however, start experimenting with alcohol and drugs, and your child may not be different. If your child has both bulimia and substance use difficulties, treatment can be considerably complicated. We have mentioned that bulimia can be quite a secretive illness, which already complicates your involvement in trying to help your child. When the eating disorder coexists with another secretive problem such as drug taking, your adolescent child will be very reluctant to have you "interfere" with any of these behaviors. You will have to approach your child very carefully under these circumstances, for you might have to follow a narrow line between convincing your teen that you want to help and antagonizing your child because she perceives you as interfering.

For youth with ARFID, comorbid psychiatric problems are the rule rather than the exception. Many will present with neurodevelopmental disorders by history, including attention-deficit/hyperactivity disorder, oppositional defiant disorder, autism spectrum disorder, posttraumatic stress disorder (PTSD), and a range of learning difficulties. For the most part these disorders are clearly present before and (with the possible exception of PTSD) will persist even after the most severe symptoms of the eating disorder are overcome. However, medications used to treat some of these disorders may have an impact on treatment and the disorder itself. Psychostimulants, antidepressants, and antipsychotics all affect appetite and weight. These factors should be carefully considered in the evaluation of any child or adolescent with ARFID.

Notwithstanding the sparse information about comorbid psychiatric illness among youth with eating disorders, if we borrow from the adult literature as well as from our own clinical experience, it seems clear that the eating disorders are indeed becoming more heterogeneous. That means there is not a "typical" adolescent with an eating disorder, and these illnesses often appear along with other psychiatric illnesses. Certainly, this makes our understanding of eating disorders more complex, and, as we've demonstrated, it inevitably complicates treatment further. A final example demonstrates this point well:

> Tina had had bulimia nervosa since she was 13 and rapidly exhibited a range of other psychiatric problems. First she became increasingly confrontational and difficult with her parents, then she began skipping school to meet boys in the park, where she smoked marijuana and drank shots. At first these activities, like her bulimia, were kept secret from her family, but over time her parents caught on. However, by that point Tina was already drinking heavily and experimenting with crack cocaine. She needed treatment in a substance abuse program before directing attention to her bulimia was even considered.

At this point there should be no doubt in your mind that eating disorders are serious illnesses that require serious attention. Think of the title of Chapter 1 as your clarion call. Go back to the warning signs and "act-now" signs listed on pages 27–28. If your child fits these descriptions, take action before an eating disorder does any more damage to your child's health. If you're concerned that your child may suffer from something other than an eating disorder, seek treatment so that these problems are prevented from doing additional harm.

It won't be easy. As you probably already know, the nature of eating disorders pits you against your child, because the eating disorder wants to stay in control. If you're to have the best possible chance of setting your child on the road to recovery quickly, you'll have to get into your child's head to get an idea of how your son or daughter actually experiences the eating disorder. Knowing how an eating disorder changes your teenager's thinking, attitudes, and behaviors will help you fight for your child's life.

FOR MORE INFORMATION

Bryant-Waugh, R. *Avoidant/Restrictive Food Intake Disorder: A Guide for Parents and Carers,* 2020. New York: Routledge.

Couturier, J., and J. Lock, Review of Medication Use for Children and Adolescents with Eating Disorders, *Journal of the Canadian Academy of Child and Adolescent Psychiatry,* 2007, *16,* 173–176.

Golden, N., D. Katzman, R. Kreipe, et al., Eating Disorders in Adolescents: Position Paper of the Society for Adolescent Medicine: Medical Indications for Hospitalization in an Adolescent with an Eating Disorder, *Journal of Adolescent Health,* 2003, *33,* 496–503.

Le Grange, D., and J. Lock, Editors, *Eating Disorders in Children and Adolescents: A Clinical Handbook,* 2011. New York: Guilford Press.

Lock, J., *The Oxford Handbook of Child and Adolescent Eating Disorders: Developmental Perspectives,* 2012. New York: Oxford University Press.

Palmer, B., *Helping People with Eating Disorders: A Clinical Guide to Assessment and Treatment,* 2000. Chichester, UK: Wiley.

Zipfel, S., B. Lowe, and W. Herzog, Medical Complications, in J. Treasure, U. Schmidt, and E. van Furth, Editors, *Handbook of Eating Disorders,* 2003. Chichester, UK: Wiley, pp. 169–190.

CHAPTER 5

Get Into Your Child's Head

The Distorted Thinking Behind Your Teenager's Behavior

If your daughter or son has an eating disorder or seems to be developing one, you've probably already been told many times, "You don't understand me" or, in fact, "Nobody understands me." This feeling is very real for someone who is struggling with an eating disorder, and it's possible that you've become very frustrated trying to understand your daughter or son. Trying to communicate your position to your troubled child can be even more problematic.

The fact is that you may *not* understand what your child is experiencing. Children and adolescents with eating disorders see their behavior—especially behavior related to food, eating, weight, exercise, and health—quite differently from the way it looks from the outside. Eating disorders alter logical ways of thinking about food and body image (except for avoidant/restrictive food intake disorder [ARFID]). They distort what your son or daughter sees in the mirror or how they feel about food and eating. They implant in your child's mind irrational expectations about the consequences of eating and not eating, exercising and not exercising.

Unless you begin to understand how your teenager's thinking has been affected by the eating disorder, your efforts to be supportive

Get Into Your Child's Head 105

of your child's struggle against the illness will be handicapped. You may be reading your child's behavior as nonsensical or defiant, when she sees perfect sense in it and is not trying to make you feel bad but hoping to make herself feel good. It may seem irrefutably clear to you that your child is emaciated and dangerously ill, but how can you hope to get her to change her behavior if you don't realize that she still sees a fat person in the mirror and feels proud of herself for sticking to her "diet"?

Your child sees herself and all things food-related through a lens imposed by the eating disorder. We call the thoughts that emerge through this lens *cognitive distortions*. In this chapter we explore the cognitive distortions that are driving your child's behavior so you can see things the way she does and thus know better how to respond constructively.

A SHIFT IN ATTITUDE, A NEW APPROACH

Before delving into specific cognitive distortions that you may be trying to deal with every day, think for a minute about the strategy you've been using in trying to resolve your teenager's disordered eating. Have you been trying to "talk some sense" into your daughter? Or are you assuming that your adolescent thinks the same way you and everyone else does when informed by common sense and reason? Now is the time to recognize that helping a child recover from an eating disorder requires, first and foremost, a new set of assumptions and a new strategy.

Understanding exactly how your child with an eating disorder is thinking is a challenge. In fact, it is often quite tricky for doctors to fully understand just how the mind of a person with anorexia nervosa, bulimia nervosa, binge-eating disorder, or ARFID works with regard to the issues of eating, weight, and dieting. Yes, you should try to develop an understanding of the ways of thinking that guide your child's behavior. But you won't always be able to fathom what makes her do what she does or feel how she feels. So the safest strategy for you as the parents to adopt is to *assume*, as hard as this may be for you, that your child's thinking with respect to weight and shape concerns and/or eating and food is probably almost always distorted. This may be especially true with anorexia nervosa.

It will also be helpful in coping with your child's illness not to underestimate just how firmly lodged these mental distortions, anxieties, and fears are. It's easy to underestimate the intransigence of these distortions, and you will often be tempted to talk some sense into your child. After all, it all seems so clear to you. Watching your child struggle to eat what appears to be a perfectly reasonable portion of food, for example, could certainly lead you to think or say, "Why not just eat it? It's so easy." Likewise, parents with a teen suffering from anorexia nervosa find themselves exhausted after lengthy and fruitless arguments, having tried to convince their child that a salad with dressing won't be harmful. The parents of someone with bulimia nervosa may discover that their child has made herself sick in the bathroom and might very well be tempted to advise her to "just stop doing it," adding, "It'll be easy; just get some self-control." For someone with a child with ARFID it is tempting to say, "Stop being so difficult and eat what's on your plate!" It is, of course, not easy at all—not for you or for your child. Eating disorders exert such a firm grip on your child's thinking that most of your pleading or arguing will be in vain.

We like to refer to such discussions as a fruitless debate with the eating disorder—parents trying, in a very rational way, to convince the child that eating is good for her or that she needs the salad or that the meal the parent so painstakingly prepared won't be harmful. Most of the time, parents lose these debates. The thinking of someone with an eating disorder is so firmly lodged in cognitive distortions and fears, there is no way you are going to argue your child out of her eating disorder. Someone with anorexia nervosa won't understand your perfectly logical argument about why this or that food item should be eaten. The beans, rice, or chicken you know will be nutritious for your child simply fills her with horror, because the food is "bad," "fattening," "unnecessary," "not the right food group," "scary," or deemed unacceptable in some other way.

When you find yourself tempted to try to reason with your child in these debates, it may help to keep one fact firmly in mind: *These cognitive distortions are at least sometimes the side effects of starvation, and dislodging such beliefs through rational debate is all but fruitless with someone who has a malnourished brain.* No doubt you were shocked by the long list of medical consequences of starvation that you read in Chapter 4. Cognitive distortions are another serious consequence, possibly the most ominous of all, because this is the one that keeps the eating disorder going. Restoring weight and normalizing eating patterns and nutrition will certainly help with this matter, but we'll get to how that happens later on.

Teenagers with bulimia nervosa have many of the same concerns about what food may "do to them" as those with anorexia nervosa. Some subtle differences may center on "forbidden foods." This is not to say that someone with anorexia nervosa would not have a long list of "forbidden foods"—quite the opposite—it's just that for those with bulimia nervosa, there are very definite foods they believe are "forbidden" because they know eating these in particular will set off a binge episode that will be followed by purging. The same is the case with binge-eating disorder, except the episode is not followed by purging, but shame and guilt nonetheless. Because this chain of events is all too familiar to your child with bulimia nervosa or binge-eating disorder, these particular foods are avoided at all costs!

COGNITIVE DISTORTIONS: HOW THINGS LOOK TO YOUR CHILD AS COMPARED WITH HOW THEY LOOK TO YOU

Accepting the fact that the eating disorder itself is making it impossible for your child to grasp reality and embrace logic in food-related matters confers a couple of important benefits:

1. It helps you separate the illness from your child and thereby remain as compassionate and empathetic as possible as you guide your child toward recovery. Interpreting refusal to eat, or denial of what the mirror declares, as defiance or some other willful negative behavior is counterproductive, only reinforcing the adversarial relationship on which the eating disorder thrives. We discuss this topic further a little later in this chapter and in Chapter 7 as well.

2. It allows you to shift your attention to exploring the specific ways in which your child thinks differently from you, which in turn will give you ideas for fighting the eating disorder in everyday situations. The rest of this chapter is devoted to the common cognitive distortions that come with eating disorders, with general suggestions for how to respond constructively. Part III of this book goes into more detail on applying this knowledge to individual situations.

It's killing her, but your daughter feels good about refusing to eat, because it's something she does well.

Youth who have eating disorders, especially those with anorexia nervosa, are usually quite driven in nature. You can't just get "a little" anorexia nervosa; you have to be "perfect" at having anorexia nervosa. In fact, you have to be better at having anorexia nervosa than anyone else with this illness. We often see girls with anorexia nervosa who, when told they need inpatient care, burst into tears in our office, saying, "But I will be the 'fattest' anorexic on the ward!" or "I can't go there—I won't be as 'good' as the others."

Youth with anorexia nervosa have usually been praised for being "determined," "focused," and "energetic," not for their anorexia nervosa, of course, but for their performance at math, cross-country, or just about anything they put their minds to. Many parents describe their teen with anorexia nervosa this way: "Once he's decided to do anything, there's no way you're going to deter him," or "When he goes for something, he gives it all he has." This quality usually leads to numerous healthy achievements in school, sports, and other extracurricular activities. The difficulty arises when everyone other than your child—you, his teachers, and his peers—recognizes these achievements, but he does not. For someone with anorexia nervosa, achievements are soon forgotten, but failures (real or perceived—getting an A– as opposed to an A+) are mulled over and quickly blot out any prior accomplishments.

This all-or-nothing thinking can be devastating. For example, Freda works very hard at being the perfect student, does her work meticulously every day, has no time to go out in the evenings or even on weekends, and has an "unblemished" report card that is a strong reminder to her that she is a "good" person and that others will like her. Without that, she'll be "nothing," "worthless," and an "utter failure." So when she was given a B in calculus, her first B ever, she was devastated. She came home sobbing, telling her parents that "things will never be the same again," "no one will ever speak to me again," and she was a "miserable failure," "dumb, stupid," and "useless!"

Often a young person with anorexia nervosa really thinks she is in fact a "loser," "good at nothing," "unattractive," and so on, when she doesn't achieve just as much as she has set out to achieve. The bar is always set high and is constantly being raised, all in an effort to convince herself that she is indeed worthy. Hilde Bruch, a famous psychoanalyst who wrote extensively about issues such as self-esteem in persons with anorexia (see Chapter 3), talked about this focus on one's failures as an "overwhelming sense of ineffectiveness."

As a result, and for reasons we don't fully understand, dieting may seem an attractive alternative solution to your child—something she thinks will "really help me feel better about myself." This may especially be the route she is attracted to when she thinks she's good at nothing else and thinks she's overweight, or someone at school or on social media made a derogatory comment about her weight, or so many other people are on diets and it seems like an admirable thing to do. Because your child has this ability to do whatever she does well, or to go all out, if she sets her mind on dieting or exercising, she will likely do these well too. Unfortunately, when she starts succeeding at dieting and/or exercise and begins losing weight, she may be encouraged by the way she looks, by the positive reinforcement she may be getting from peers or from her family, by her improved performance at cross-country running, and so on. It seems easy then for this achievement to supplant most other achievements, and it soon becomes the only thing your child thinks she does well.

In fact, anorexia nervosa is often associated with an immense sense of pride: "I can say 'no' to food when everyone else does not have such willpower" or "I can lose weight successfully when all of you are struggling just to shed a pound" or "I can run this extra mile even though I have not eaten much all day—none of you would be able to do that." This sense of "better than you" might be subtle, but if it's the only thing your teen thinks she's good at, she will do everything to defend it. Thus, soon this ability to go without food is seen as her only sense of accomplishment, and anyone who attempts to persuade her to gain weight is seen as ignorant at best, but most likely as cruel and insensitive. It therefore feels incongruous when others criticize the teenager for being such a successful dieter (something many peers and parents have failed at) or try to "derail" his twice-daily routine of 200 crunches, 200 push-ups, 200 sit-ups, and so on. Your child feels that others are simply envious.

Again, the struggle for most parents is tackling this relentlessness that is so characteristic of eating disorders, without feeling as if they are taking something perceived to be so precious away from their child. Indeed, most youth with anorexia nervosa will make parents feel as if they're being most unkind in getting them to gain weight, while the parents will have to find a way to persevere in their efforts to help their child redirect her ability to be a "good anorexic" into another, much more fruitful and healthier endeavor.

Your child's behavior demonstrates that she's out of control, but she sees it as a way to stay in charge and express her independence.

In the usual pursuit of autonomy, there are many ways in which adolescents seek control of their own lives: choosing their own friends, driving themselves where they need to go, setting their own standards of performance, and so on. However, when adolescents' choices indicate they are not in control—binge drinking, serious risk-taking behavior, *and* anorexia and bulimia nervosa, to name just a few examples—the issue for parents is clearly how to set appropriate limits on independence and control. When dieting leads to anorexia nervosa, the adolescent needs help to reestablish normal adolescent autonomy processes and experimentation, and the options available do not include food restriction or overexercise. The same is true when food restriction leads to bouts of binge eating, whether followed by purging or not. Parents often have to assist youth in normalizing eating (for example, three healthy meals per day and several snacks) so that other aspects of adolescent experimentation do not also suffer as a consequence of the lack of healthy eating patterns.

The challenge for most parents, though, is that although the child's behavior demonstrates that she is out of control, she will more than likely see the eating disorder as the only way to stay in charge and express some independence. She will vigorously fend off any attempts you might make to help. There will be little you can do that won't be perceived as "you're always telling me what to do" or "you always want to control my every move."

Anorexia nervosa may look somewhat different from bulimia nervosa or binge-eating disorder in some respects. Youth with anorexia nervosa will probably come across as quite "together" or "in control" of their lives. In fact, the illness is often associated with a great sense of order, neatness, and discipline. Grades in school continue to be high. All this serves to confuse most parents as they contemplate the fact that their child is perhaps not in charge of things. We've often heard parents say, "Yes, she's 17 and weighs 82 pounds, but her grades are excellent, she's really working hard, and she's doing so well." The dilemma is made even more difficult by the fact that your daughter with anorexia nervosa will assert, repeatedly, that she is fine, that she is in control, and that she can make her own decisions in a rational way. Your daughter will be so persuasive in her arguments that you will find it hard not to believe her. The irony is that the illness also has the ability to convince her that she is indeed in charge of her eating and weight management, and that she can stop dieting and losing weight anytime she wants—"just not now!"

"I can take care of this myself" is also very persuasive to most parents, frightened about what they think might happen to their child but desperate in their willingness to believe that she can get better by herself, as she's repeatedly assured them she can. However, the way the physiology and psychology of starvation work is that at a certain point, usually once weight loss has clearly begun, the child loses control over this process and cannot stop dieting, or get herself to eat a decent amount of food, even if she *wants* to. The anorexia nervosa has firmly established its own control over the thinking and behavior of your adolescent.

This is a critical point to remember at all times: *Once your child has reached the point of significant preoccupation with and actual weight loss, she often cannot get better by herself, even if she proclaims that she can.*

As a parent, you need to realize that this doesn't necessarily mean she does not want to get better. It's just that the anorexia nervosa is more powerful as an illness than your child's solo efforts at defeating the illness. Remember your new set of assumptions when you're tempted to fall back into the attitude that your child is just being obstinate and all it will take for her to start eating normally again is for you to talk some sense into her.

Again, the only way to get your child out of this dilemma is for you and her treatment team to help her restore her weight. *It is only with normalization of eating behaviors and weight restoration when needed that she will be able to think in healthy and rational ways, and it is only with these improvements that she will have a chance to get back on track with a normal developmental trajectory and achieve healthy and appropriate control over her individuation and budding independence.*

Bulimia nervosa and binge-eating disorder are not altogether different, but with these illnesses it may be easier for you to notice that your adolescent is indeed out of control. You can probably think of many times that you've missed a box of cookies from the pantry: You knew it was there just this morning, and now it's gone. You remember putting last night's leftover chicken in the fridge, and now it's missing. You've noticed the candy wrappers in the trash in Maggie's room every day! And in the case of bulimia nervosa, you've also spotted the remnants of her purging in the bathroom, week after week now.

Many young people with bulimia nervosa or binge-eating disorder may feel ambivalent about anyone interfering with their attempts to control their weight, their eating, and even their purging, but are in fact often quite relieved when a parent helps them succeed in breaking the shameful pattern of binge eating and/or purging. Another difference in bulimia nervosa and binge-eating disorder, as compared with anorexia nervosa, is a youth with bulimia nervosa will not so stridently insist that she is in control of her eating. In fact, every time she has a binge-eating or purging episode, your daughter feels more and more out of control: "I feel disgusted with myself every time I do this, but I just don't know how to stop." In the case of bulimia nervosa, this is followed by thoughts such as "I am so afraid that I will gain weight if I don't make myself sick, and that's why I just can't stop doing this." However, some youth may deny feeling out of control, especially as they'll probably make every effort to reestablish control over eating *after* a binge/purge episode. Unlike with anorexia nervosa, this sense of control seldom lasts for more than a couple of days, only to be followed by binge eating and, in the case of bulimia nervosa, purging again. Nevertheless, your daughter with bulimia nervosa or binge-eating disorder is probably more likely to assert that she is, in fact, in control of her behavior and that it isn't up to you to tell her what to do about her difficulties. This is particularly confusing to you as a parent, as you've seen your child acting quite independently in so many other areas of her adolescence. Helping her with her bulimia nervosa or binge-eating disorder may now seem almost counterintuitive!

Whether your child has anorexia nervosa, bulimia nervosa, or binge-eating disorder, it is highly likely that he won't think he is out of control and will probably resent you for trying to help. The challenge for you is how you will delicately balance your understanding of your child's developmental need for independence with your understanding of his dilemma and find a way to help him assert healthy control over his life at a time when he might resent you for your "interference." What is clear, though, is that you don't really have a choice. You have to help your child as the eating disorder continues to cloud his judgment.

To you, this is a deadly disease; to your child with anorexia, it's "just a perfectly healthy diet."

You now realize just how devastating an eating disorder is, but to see your child being flippant about her low heart rate, anemia, blood in her vomit, and swollen parotid glands is to come face-to-face with one of the most alarming aspects of anorexia and bulimia—the inability of the person with the eating disorder to appreciate just how deadly these illnesses can be. This denial of the seriousness of the severe malnutrition associated with anorexia nervosa is a core symptom of the illness. Teens with bulimia nervosa or binge-eating disorder will not necessarily understand the seriousness of their symptoms either, especially the long-term serious health consequences. Someone with anorexia does not appreciate how lethal severe emaciation can be, and similarly, someone with bulimia does not understand that low potassium, due to frequent vomiting, for instance, can cause death. For those with binge-eating disorder, the risk of obesity, diabetes, and hypertension may seem remote. Still, it's fair to say that this denial is more pronounced in anorexia.

In Chapter 4 we explained that anorexia is an ego-syntonic illness. What this means is that, unlike those with many other mental disorders, the patient with anorexia "likes" or "cherishes" the illness or "takes comfort" in it. Someone with anorexia doesn't appreciate its dangers and will do almost anything to protect it, that is, prevent you from "taking it away." Although parents and doctors alike find this aspect of anorexia very difficult to understand, it helps to think of anorexia in comparison with other mental disorders: The patient who is depressed wants to feel better, the person who is anxious wants to relax, but the person with anorexia still wants to be thinner. This denial is actually reinforced through constant dieting and further weight loss, as well as focusing on these issues (dieting and weight) all the time to the exclusion of other, healthier perspectives. Thus, her diet is still normal to your daughter, even though everyone else sees it for what it is. Therefore, it's not uncommon for someone with anorexia to take pride in brushes with death: "Wow, I got my potassium down to 1.8, and I made it." (Showing up in the emergency room with a potassium level that low is considered most critical, and few people can be revived.)

What makes this illness so incredibly dangerous is that no matter how much you argue this very point with your teenager with anorexia—"You could have died. . . . We are so lucky they managed to revive you at the hospital. . . . We were so, so scared. . . . Do you understand how serious this is?"—these facts usually will have little impact on your son. Quietly, your teen will perceive this "crisis" as another achievement in his quest for that ideal weight.

By comparison, bulimia and binge-eating disorder are more ego-dystonic. What this means is that although an adolescent with bulimia or binge-eating disorder exhibits many of the aspects of denial of her illness that are common in anorexia, there is less pride involved in her symptoms. Rather, great discomfort and shame are associated with binge eating and purging. Nevertheless, this doesn't mean that your son or daughter will be forthcoming and ask for help as an adolescent who is depressed or anxious might. Quite the opposite is true. Because thinness is highly valued and the seriousness of the illness is not appreciated, *and* because of the guilt and shame associated with binge eating, most adolescents will do their best to binge eat without your knowledge. For those with bulimia, the anxiety that the food they ate will make them gain 5 pounds overnight is so overwhelming that they absolutely "have to" get rid of it and will make every effort to make sure there's a way to purge after the binge-eating episodes. It certainly is not uncommon for a teenager with bulimia to evaluate an invitation for a movie and a meal with her friends based not on what movie they'll see or what kind of food (Asian, Italian, Mexican) they'll eat, but rather on the answers to questions such as "Will I be able to purge at that restaurant?" or "Can I slip away at that movie theater to use the bathroom to throw up?"

Thinking, Fears, and Disgust in ARFID

Youth with ARFID have concerns and worries that differ from those that characterize anorexia nervosa, bulimia nervosa, and binge-eating disorder. These concerns are not focused on weight and shape, but instead are serious cognitive and emotional reactions to food and eating that lead to social, nutritional, and developmental impairments. The child who is "too busy" to eat, is never hungry, and whines at every meal when encouraged to eat enough to grow and have metabolic health is not willfully disobedient, though it may seem that way to parents who are worried about him. Instead, he feels "forced" to eat when he feels no hunger, making him frustrated by being told what to do and failing to recognize his need for nutrition. Similarly, the child who is afraid that if she eats she will choke, not be able to breathe, and maybe die is not being melodramatic. Her fear is genuine and disorganizing her emotional life and relationships with others, especially her parents, who are frightened for her health. Fear—whether in anorexia nervosa or in the context of ARFID—is a very powerful emotion, so much so that in response a person will do almost anything to avoid experiencing it. Avoiding fear leads to avoiding eating, and avoiding eating leads to malnutrition. You child does not choose to be afraid—they are trying not to be afraid—but they are afraid of being afraid.

For those who have ARFID as a result of extreme picky eating, it is not fear so much as anticipation of feeling disgusted that motivates their limited food choices. Disgust is a powerful response that has both emotional and cognitive dimensions. Disgust is likely a biologically based response that helps protect us from poisonous or harmful foods. Similarly, sensitivity to tastes and textures vary significantly from person and person—one person may like hot sauce and another cannot bear it—and these sensitivities have both biological and social origins. So, when your child has an extremely limited range of foods in his diet, it is important to remember that disgust and food taste and texture sensitivities are not really your child's choice but rather his response to foods he finds disgusting (or appear likely to be so). Trying to argue with your child about these responses to eating leads to frustration on all sides.

As has probably become clear by now, gaining a better understanding of how the eating disorder leads your child to think and behave in very fixed ways concerning weight, shape, and eating issues will be helpful to you in finding the right way to help your adolescent overcome this struggle. That doesn't mean this understanding will automatically suggest an instantly effective strategy; it's just that without this understanding you're unlikely even to know why your efforts fail. Chapters 7 and 8 offer various ideas for helping your child, based on your understanding of these cognitive distortions.

You're the enemy, even though you're trying to save your son's life, because you're "forcing" him to do the one thing he is trying to avoid: eat.

The cognitive distortions and emotional reaction borne of eating disorders, by their very nature, create an adversarial relationship between you and your child. You want your child to eat appropriately to regain his health; he is firmly committed to continuing to lose weight or to hiding the truth that he is binge eating and purging or continuing to eat the same four things that he feels comfortable consuming. The fact that you can't "talk some sense into him" means that any attempt you make to confront your child's false beliefs and consequent denial only makes you seem like a greater enemy.

The rift between you may seem to widen from your own perspective too when you try to confront your child about irrational beliefs surrounding food and weight. You may very well have come to count on the rational discussion and sharing of decision making that are among the beneficial developments of life with an adolescent. In fact, you may feel today that you have a perfectly rational person around the house most of the time—"We can talk about homework, our vacation plans, or the music she likes to listen to"—but when it comes to food, eating, and weight issues, "it's as if a switch was turned off; she makes no sense, and the worst is, she doesn't see the difference." The fact that your child is no longer meeting your expectations for rationality may make you feel as if it's the child who is creating the adversarial situation. With this kind of standoff, who wins?

The eating disorder wins.

That's because the real—and only—enemy is the anorexia nervosa, bulimia nervosa, binge-eating disorder, or ARFID. Recognizing this is the key to responding constructively to these powerful emotional responses and cognitive distortions.

The concerns associated with eating disorders can be so severe that rational discussion and decision sharing about your child's health are no longer possible. Parents have to be prepared to accept the idea that in the areas of food, eating, and weight, they are no longer dealing with a child who is rational. It is the *illness* they are dealing with.

We've seen many parents in distress when their usually kind child lashes out when the parents make any attempt to intervene in the illness: "I don't want to eat that! You're killing me. Can't you see how unhappy you make me?" or "I hate you, I want nothing to do with you, don't even talk to me!" or "Leave me alone! You are making me *so* miserable." Desperate utterances from your child sounding anything like these are obviously distressing to any parent. What the young person with an eating disorder wants is for you to back off in your efforts to help. As tempting as this might be for many parents, acquiescing only means allowing the illness to triumph.

What can you do? Negotiating with your child under these circumstances is a great challenge and one that you are most likely to lose. In defense of his illness, your son will try to make sure that your efforts fail, whether you are trying to get him to eat more or to keep him from purging the food that he has consumed. Knowing that there is little you can do to rationally argue, discuss, or convince your son about the perils of his illness and that the behaviors he is manifesting are illness related as opposed to those of "your child" (separating the illness from your adolescent) will help you when you're trying to help him. Knowing that getting involved in "eating disorder debates" will be fruitless and that you will probably lose the argument and end up being convinced, against your own better judgment, that an apple is better than a pasta dish with a cream sauce for a starving teenager, it's best not to argue. Instead, you will want to find a way to let your child know that you understand his dilemma, that the illness doesn't allow him to be rational about food and weight right now, that you understand that for the time being he sees you as the enemy, but that none of this can deter you from doing what you know will save his life—to get him to eat what he should eat to be healthy and/or to keep him from binge eating and purging.

Earlier we mentioned the concept of separating the illness from your adolescent. This is an important principle in dealing with a teenager with an eating disorder, just as it is in helping someone of any age with any psychiatric disorder. Understanding how the illness is "separate" from your child will be crucial in helping you understand your child's troubled behaviors and deal with the illness effectively. We discuss this principle in more detail in Chapter 7.

"Not eating" is not just the most important thing in the life of your daughter with anorexia nervosa: It's "the only thing."

For parents, it is often very difficult to understand just how important eating or not eating, weight loss, or feeling the "right" size is to their child. In fact, for someone with anorexia nervosa, nothing can be more important than focusing on that next pound to lose or making sure not to eat at all until 5:00 P.M. every day of the next week. For someone with bulimia nervosa, nothing can be more important than how she can get rid of the food she has just eaten, believing it's going to make her fat. Indeed, managing to adhere to all these "rules" and "regulations" around eating or not eating eventually eclipses the importance of school, family, and friends, or at least it appears to do so, especially if the eating disorder behaviors are allowed to continue unchecked. It is especially hard for parents to witness their kind child appear completely oblivious to other crises in the family—it's not uncommon for a person with anorexia nervosa to show little concern for a parent who was just diagnosed with a severe illness, because she is so preoccupied with the quest for thinness. This young person is, of course, not heartless; it's just that eating disorders have a way of overtaking the sufferer, leaving little room for anything else.

Paradoxically, when someone with anorexia nervosa continues to starve himself, it actually becomes easier and easier not to eat. At the onset of the illness the young person has to work very hard to keep his appetite "in check," making sure he doesn't "give in" to these "horrible urges" to eat, always feeling that he cannot let his guard down for a moment. With increasing weight loss, though, it becomes easier to feel a sense of mastery over these urges, and with time the young person no longer feels any hunger. However, with increased starvation, he also becomes more preoccupied with thoughts about food and weight. In fact, some young people find themselves in the unenviable position where they can think of virtually nothing else but "What is that half bagel from this morning going to do to my weight?" or "What can I do to avoid having lunch with my friends?" or "How can I make sure that I have no more than a salad without dressing for dinner?" and so on. It's hard to imagine just how much of their time, on a daily basis, will be taken up by such thoughts. Some teens with anorexia will say, "I can think of nothing else but my weight—literally nothing else!"

Much of what happens with the dieting adolescent, especially when starvation has set in, also happens to people who lose extreme amounts of weight because of a variety of medical illnesses. In fact, much of what we know about the effects of starvation on the human mind and on human behavior is derived from what we have learned from individuals without an eating disorder. Ancel Keys and his colleagues, in a landmark study in Minnesota in the early 1950s, published their results of a semi-starvation study of World War II conscientious objectors. The physical and psychological changes in these healthy men who were starved for several months were the same as those we typically observe in our patients with an eating disorder—the men became increasingly preoccupied with their weight and with food once they had lost a substantial amount of weight. It's almost as if the part of the brain that controls hunger and satiety will not let you forget about the one thing you need most when you're starved—food! The good news is that once these starved study participants were allowed to eat normally again, their weights were restored and the symptoms of starvation also disappeared. These observations reveal exactly what we also witness in many patients with anorexia when they return to a healthy weight.

Your daughter with anorexia nervosa has consumed mere crumbs of food, but she thinks she's telling the truth when she says she's eaten a huge amount of food today.

When your child has consumed only a few bites of her sandwich and proclaims to have eaten "tons" or "too much" or a "huge amount," there are at least two ways in which her account is accurate from her perspective. First, she sees eating anything at all as a failure and a sign of weakness. So, psychologically, even a small amount is the same as a large amount to her. The anxiety and guilt she experiences after eating half a bagel are the same as if she had eaten a whole sandwich. Second, and in reality, the stomach of someone with anorexia nervosa usually decreases in capacity, and as a consequence, the rate at which the stomach empties has been slowed. It's therefore quite likely that your child will feel full and stay feeling that way longer after eating even a relatively small amount of food. Moreover, prolonged starvation has allowed your child's hunger cues to be stilled, making eating even more difficult when she states that she's not hungry. So, when she does eat, even what are in fact mere crumbs, your daughter will feel that she has overeaten on both accounts. "I will get fat if I eat that bagel (half an apple/three carrots/and so on)," she will say, or "I just can't eat that much, I've already had enough," in reference to the small bowl of salad without dressing that sits half eaten. These incidents are, in fact, experienced by your child as really having eaten too much or really finding it hard to eat the "whole" salad.

The situation is further complicated when parents want to believe their child's account of what was eaten when they (the parents) weren't around to supervise a meal. And parents can become increasingly despondent when their child doesn't gain weight despite "all the food" she claims to be eating on a regular basis. It is very important for you to remember that eating even half an apple at school lunch, when your child has promised himself (though really promised his anorexia nervosa) not to eat at all, is seen by him as a calamitous transgression of crucial food rules and that the half apple was a huge amount of food—"huge" because it "should not have been eaten." Likewise, asking your child to tell you what she ate for lunch at school might get you a response along these lines: "A yogurt and an apple and a milkshake." That may sound like enough, but if you inquire carefully, it may in fact mean that in reality she ate a scoop of yogurt, ate a bite of an apple, and had a sip of a milkshake. As has become clear to you by now, even when your child protests about "too much food" or says, "I can't possibly have more to eat," recovery from anorexia can really come about only when sufficiently healthy amounts of food are consumed to return your child's thinking about these issues to normal and, of course, to restore gut functioning to normal.

The same scenario may be true for an adolescent with bulimia nervosa or binge-eating disorder, but it will take a slightly different form. Whereas your child who binge eats will also try to restrict her food intake and may also consider mere crumbs of food "a lot," many young people who binge eat are very scared that if they eat "one more crumb" than their self-imposed food rules allow, they will "just go ahead and eat the whole cake." Sadly, that is what happens for young people who binge eat, and that's why your child will so rigidly try to hang on to these beliefs.

No matter how emaciated she becomes, what your daughter with anorexia nervosa sees in the mirror is a fat person.

This is called *body image distortion*, which is a result of an overfocus on weight and shape that eventually leads to misapprehension of realities. Many young people with anorexia nervosa overestimate their own body size, and quite paradoxically, the thinner they become, the more they may see themselves as fat. Body image distortion is much less common among those with bulimia nervosa, binge-eating disorder, or ARFID. In the case of bulimia nervosa and binge-eating disorder, instead of body image distortion per se, there is an overvaluation of appearance, especially related to weight. Some youth with eating disorders may go so far as to cover all mirrors in their homes so that they can never catch a glimpse of themselves.

Unfortunately, the only "solution" the young person can think of to escape this agonizing dilemma is to lose yet another pound, thereby establishing a cycle of further weight loss and further distortion of reality. One insightful young person with anorexia nervosa described her experience like this: "I thought I was fat when I wore these pants. Now that I have gained weight I can't see any difference (I still look as fat), but the pants are the same. I guess I can't see things the way they really are. My fear of being fat makes me look fat no matter what." Many young people, though, know they are thin and don't actually see themselves as fat, yet they still cannot escape "feeling fat." Someone might say, "I know I'm not fat, but every morning I wake up feeling fat, and I know there's only one way to tackle my problem and that's to lose more weight. Perhaps then I won't feel fat." What may be happening here for some young people who are predisposed to developing an eating disorder is that it's "easier" to wake up in the morning and focus on their weight than to think about "that issue at school" or "the breakup with my boyfriend." Many teenagers with eating disorders may not know how to tackle or resolve the issues that cause them to feel depressed or anxious, but it's a little "easier" to go on a diet and lose weight. So, instead of waking up saying "I am depressed" or "I am anxious" and then having to figure out how to deal with that feeling, it seems somewhat more manageable to "replace" the depression or anxiety with "I feel fat," because at least "I have a plan to cut back on my food intake some more and lose another pound. Maybe then I'll feel okay."

Obviously, losing that extra pound does not help with the feeling of fatness. But even with that evidence before her—that losing an extra pound doesn't eliminate her feeling of being fat—you will find it very difficult, if not impossible, to convince your child that she isn't fat. As long as that "feeling" persists, the young person will stay on the cycle of trying to lose weight, and not eating will continue to cause the body image distortion that tells her loud and clear that she is fat. Body image distortion usually, but not always, improves or even normalizes after weight has been restored for a period of a few months in an outpatient setting.

Your son with bulimia nervosa continues to vomit even though his weight is clearly increasing.

One of the ironies of bulimia nervosa is that the weight-control strategy of purging is quite ineffective. It is impossible to vomit up the full amount one has eaten during an hour-long binge-eating episode—too much food has already entered the intestinal tract. Thus, a hefty percentage of these high-calorie foods remains in the system and adds weight. Over time, then, instead of losing weight, patients with bulimia nervosa tend to gain weight. However, this only adds to the urgency of their efforts to control their weight, which leads to increasing self-starvation, binge eating, and then purging. Still, they keep on doing it. Why?

The answer is, in part, that over time binge eating and purging are experienced as a coping strategy for life's other problems. Over time, young people report feeling tremendous relief after purging. This reinforces the purging behaviors whether or not they lead to weight loss. Many people who have been ill for a while readily admit that they know the purging does little to help them with weight control: "It's just that I have to do it. I feel much better afterward, even if that feeling doesn't last very long." So, when your son feels he didn't perform well at a wrestling meet, he may binge eat and purge. The same is true when your daughter breaks up with her boyfriend or is having academic trouble. In other words, binge eating and purging are no longer efforts at weight control alone; they are also used more generally in an effort to cope with other problems. When a behavior like binge eating and purging is being used to manage life's other problems, it's harder to let go of, and the "logic" that it doesn't control weight doesn't pertain.

Your daughter seems prideful about her self-starvation but miserable at the same time.

One of the hardest things to appreciate about severe dieting is that although your child appears to be reveling in the accomplishment of lower and lower weights, she is also quite miserable. Anorexia nervosa is a very tough taskmaster. Whenever your child eats even a small amount, she experiences severe harassing and critical thoughts about failure and worthlessness. These thoughts are unrelenting and merciless. In addition, the preoccupation with eating, obsessive and repetitive thinking about how much was eaten and how many calories were consumed, weight gain, and so forth disrupt usual thinking, making it sometimes difficult to focus in school or during social gatherings. The point is, however determined and steadfast your child appears, she is really suffering, physically and psychologically, as a result of the punitive thinking experienced.

Young people with bulimia nervosa are usually filled with shame and feelings of failure because they "give in" to eating and "purge" even though it's disgusting. These adolescents experience a combination of guilt, shame, recrimination, and anxiety about gaining weight. It helps to have a sympathetic view of this experience, because as a parent, when your child is suffering, you want to relieve that suffering, even if the illness behaviors are themselves frustrating and provoke anger in you.

Children with ARFID often feel they are a disappointment to their parents—they feel that if they eat when they are afraid, disgusted, or not hungry they will be miserable, but if they do as their

Get Into Your Child's Head

parents ask, they will feel uncomfortable, feel overwhelmed, or have extremely unpleasant eating experiences. They are stuck between a rock and a hard place. Consequently, they are sometimes oppositional, angry, tearful, and defiant in the face of parental requests to eat more and/or differently. Parents who understand these feelings and react to them with compassion, while also not allowing their child to continue undereating or eating a completely unhealthy diet, will be more successful in the long run at helping their child manage and recover from ARFID.

Your son weighs himself 10 times a day and is constantly pinching himself to see if he has any fat despite his obvious severe weight loss.

Body checking and repeated weighing appear irrational to us because we know that weight does not vary much during a single day and that pinching or repeatedly checking our appearance in the mirror will not provide new information. However, the anxiety about weight gain and a concomitant hyperfocus on body fat are pervasive in young people with anorexia nervosa, bulimia nervosa, and binge-eating disorder. To combat perceived weight gain or actual but needed weight gain, those with these eating disorders look for reassurance in these constant "checking" activities, whether it's pinching the stomach or thighs a hundred times a day or standing in front of the mirror for what seems like hours at a time, checking and rechecking to see whether any weight was put on. Unfortunately, the reassurance is only momentary (if at all), and they quickly need to check again. If you remember that these behaviors also reinforce the hyperfocus on shape and weight concerns, you will see why it's often necessary to find ways to help your child reduce his dependence on such strategies so as to reduce his anxiety about weight and shape. For instance, you might make this struggle a great deal easier for your child if you remove your bathroom scale. You can reassure your child that he will be weighed at regular intervals at the doctor's office, and it is at the doctor's office that these concerns can be addressed.

Your daughter promises to stop binge eating, but every day you find missing food cartons and potato chip bags under her bed.

Your daughter's intentions to stop binge eating are sincere and genuine. She wishes she could follow through on them. It is not a loss of willpower or a character problem or just wanting to be spiteful. Rather, it is that she has learned to use food to manage her emotions, conflicts, and self-esteem. Food is very reinforcing for most of us (though not—as we have noted—for some children with **ARFID**) because it is immediately rewarding on a physical and neurochemical level. Food has also been used to soothe, comfort, and reward in socially condoned ways throughout history and currently. Your daughter may not care about the long-term effects of binge eating on her weight or health, but the short-term rewards are hard to ignore, especially when she is feeling overwhelmed and doesn't have an alternative strategy to help her cope.

WHAT'S A PARENT SUPPOSED TO DO?

When you understand your child's thinking with regard to the emotional and cognitive problems we've discussed, you've laid the foundation for whatever practical interventions you will implement to help fight your child's eating disorder. By separating the illness from your child (also called *externalizing the illness*), you support your child as a developing young person while insisting that she fight the eating disorder nonetheless.

As we've shown, eating disorders are clearly very complicated illnesses, both in terms of the effects of starvation and maladaptive eating and eating patterns on the mind and the body, and in terms of how coexisting psychiatric illnesses further complicate the picture. In addition, as we've seen in this chapter, how your child experiences the effects makes her thinking and behaviors appear irrational and confusing, though there is a kind of logic when you understand them better.

Treatment for eating disorders must respond to these complicated thoughts, behaviors, and, at times, medical problems. What this usually means is that good treatment pays attention to all aspects of these illnesses—psychological, psychiatric, medical, and nutritional. Good treatment also means that you, the parent, play an active role in helping your child receive care and that you actively participate in this care. Your involvement in treatment is particularly helpful here, as these emotional and cognitive distortions are so persistent and so powerful that someone has to be on hand to help counteract them, and, obviously, the parents (and the rest of the family) are usually the only ones routinely in the position to do this.

In the following chapter, we outline what research to date has been able to tell us about the effectiveness of the best-studied treatments for eating disorders. If you choose to have family therapy along the lines of FBT (see Chapter 7), it will help you use everything you now know about how your child thinks to enhance your success in taking charge of the problematic eating behavior. If you choose among other types of treatment, you can still use what you know about emotional and cognitive distortions to support the treatment team's efforts, as described in Chapter 8.

FOR MORE INFORMATION

Bryant-Waugh, R. *Avoidant/Restrictive Food Intake Disorder: A Guide for Parents and Carers*, 2020. New York: Routledge.

Le Grange, D., and J. Lock, Editors, *Eating Disorders in Children and Adolescents: A Clinical Handbook*, 2011. New York: Guilford Press.

Lock, J., *The Oxford Handbook of Child and Adolescent Eating Disorders: Developmental Perspectives*, 2012. New York: Oxford University Press.

Treasure, J., and B. Bauer, Assessment and Motivation, in J. Treasure, U. Schmidt, and E. van Furth, Editors, *Handbook of Eating Disorders*, 2003. Chichester, UK: Wiley, pp. 219–232.

CHAPTER 6

Understand Your Options

What the Research Says about the Best Ways to Treat Anorexia Nervosa, Bulimia Nervosa, Binge-Eating Disorder, and Avoidant/Restrictive Food Intake Disorder

Having a better understanding of your adolescent's difficulties involving self-esteem, body weight, shape, and eating habits enables you to take the next step: finding help. Identifying the most appropriate treatment for your child can be a challenge, however, because researchers and the clinical community still struggle with many unknowns. Fortunately, we know more today than ever before about treatments that reverse self-starvation or binge eating and purging, and normalize eating in children with avoidant/restrictive food intake disorder (ARFID), which can assist you and your child in understanding some of the psychological makeup of her difficulties and help get your child back on track with her developmental trajectory.

In this chapter we present what we know about the different treatments for eating disorders. Before we get into the specifics, however, it's important to understand that most treatment studies providing evidence for the effectiveness of these therapies have focused exclusively on people who meet the full criteria for an eating disorder. This does not mean that no treatment is available if your child does not meet the full criteria for an eating disorder. Clinical experience has shown that in most settings a child whose symptoms resemble those of people with an eating disorder should be treated the same way those who meet the full criteria for these disorders are treated. And in some ways, the outcome might be more favorable for your child if she has been ill for only a few months or a year and does not qualify for the full diagnosis of a specific eating disorder. *An important point to remember as you read about the available treatment options is that early and good treatment usually bodes well for your child's recovery from an eating disorder.* We start by discussing studies that evaluate outpatient approaches, and we then turn to more intensive therapies such as inpatient, day-hospital, or residential treatments.

OUTPATIENT TREATMENTS

In this section we explain what the latest research has shown about the effectiveness of the main psychological treatments for eating disorders (family therapy, psychodynamic individual therapy, cognitive-behavioral therapy, interpersonal psychotherapy, and nutritional counseling) and medication treatments.

Psychological Treatments

Anorexia Nervosa. Only a few treatments for youth with anorexia nervosa have been studied systematically using valid scientific methods. Psychological treatments for anorexia nervosa that have been studied include family-based treatment (FBT), adolescent-focused therapy (AFT), and cognitive-behavioral therapy (CBT). Ten randomized clinical trials with a total of 1,008 adolescent participants have evaluated FBT. In these studies, FBT was either as effective as or superior to comparison therapies, and FBT also worked more quickly in promoting weight gain and decreased the need for hospitalization. More recent studies have shown that FBT can be effective in different formats: a parent-only format, sometimes called separated family therapy or parent-focused therapy (PFT); or FBT delivered online, in multifamily groups, or in a guided self-help (GSH) program. Other studies have explored whether FBT for anorexia nervosa could be useful for older adolescents and young adults—transition-age youth. The results of these studies, while not definitive, suggest that FBT is helpful for many young people in the slightly older age group. These developments allow the reach of FBT to be extended to families where all family members cannot participate or live too far away from treatment centers to attend in-person therapy, and to regions where there are few trained clinicians in FBT. Most recently, a study confirmed that the addition of a few sessions (intensive parental coaching) focused on improving parental effectiveness at refeeding was helpful for families who felt particularly ineffective before starting FBT and whose child failed to gain much weight during the first few sessions of FBT.

An alternative to FBT is AFT. This is an individual therapy aimed at addressing adolescent self-efficacy and autonomy. It has been studied in two randomized clinical trials and in both was not as effective as family therapy, but nonetheless promoted significant clinical progress in many participants. In examining who did better in AFT, it appears that youth who were overall less symptomatic did better. That is, adolescents who were less obsessional about their eating, who did not purge in the context of anorexia, and whose eating-related cognitions were not as pronounced appeared to do well in AFT.

CBT for anorexia nervosa was developed based on an approach developed for adults with bulimia nervosa. Studies of adults with anorexia nervosa using CBT demonstrated that it was a more cost-effective approach compared to treatment as usual or hospitalization. A recent study using an enhanced version of CBT (CBT-E) in adults with anorexia nervosa found that it was helpful for some, but the overall response was not impressive. Other studies of adults with anorexia nervosa comparing CBT-E found no difference in outcome among randomized treatment groups and most patients were still significantly ill. Research on CBT-E with adolescents is limited, but several nonrandomized studies conducted in specialized treatment centers found significant improvements in weight and cognitions over time. Thus, CBT-E for children and adolescents with anorexia nervosa may best be described at this time as a potentially effective

Understand Your Options

approach that requires further systematic study (including randomized comparison treatments and different study sites) before it can be called an effective treatment for the disorder in this age group.

Bulimia Nervosa. Although there have been a number of treatment studies for the treatment of adults with bulimia nervosa, there have been only four randomized clinical trials that examined treatments for adolescents with bulimia nervosa. One study compared a version of family therapy to a therapist-supported self-help version of CBT. It found that adolescents did about the same in both treatments. The second study compared FBT to an individual supportive therapy and found that those in family therapy improved more quickly and did better overall. Another large randomized clinical trial compared CBT to usual care in child mental health programs in the United Kingdom. This study found no differences between the two, but CBT did lead to clinical improvements in terms of weight and cognitions in those treated using it. This most recent study was a relatively large clinical trial with 136 adolescents, randomized to either FBT or CBT, that found FBT was more effective at the end of 6 months of treatment, but that patients in CBT continued to improve during follow-up and "caught up" statistically with those in FBT. Thus it appears that FBT is faster in promoting improvements in bulimia nervosa and is thereby usually recognized as the preferred treatment in guidelines.

While there are no other treatment studies of youth with bulimia nervosa, studies of adults have been done on interpersonal psychotherapy (IPT), a treatment that focuses on the role of difficulties in relationships in eating disorder symptoms, and dialectical behavior therapy (DBT), a treatment that focuses on learning how to manage emotions. A study that compared IPT to CBT found that CBT worked more quickly, but over time there were no differences in outcome between the two treatments. DBT is effective for adults with bulimia nervosa and adolescents with problems of suicidal ideation and self-injury. Some therapists are using DBT with adolescent patients who have bulimia nervosa and suicidal ideation or thoughts of self-injury, but how effective this treatment will be is not yet known.

Binge-Eating Disorder. Many studies have been done on the treatment of binge-eating disorder in adults. These studies suggest that this disorder responds to many treatments, including CBT, IPT, and DBT. For youth with binge-eating disorders, IPT has been used in a number of patients, but no randomized clinical trials have been reported. However, FBT studies of bulimia nervosa suggest effectiveness of the approach for binge-eating behaviors in youth and therefore it too should be considered as a possibly efficacious treatment for this age group.

Avoidant/Restrictive Food Intake Disorder. There are two treatments that have been studied for ARFID in youth. FBT for ARFID has been reported effective in case series data, with noted improvements in range of foods eaten and weight gain in underweight children. A small randomized clinical trial compared FBT to treatment as usual and found FBT was more effective. CBT has also been studied in several case series reports on older children, adolescents, and young adults and demonstrated improvement in symptoms of ARFID and weight gain. Both FBT and CBT are potentially effective treatments for youth with ARFID, but both require further systematic study to demonstrate efficacy and effectiveness. In clinical practice, therapists develop individualized behavior plans that provide rewards for changes in behavior, usually by gradually increasing food intake in terms of both types of food and amounts. Parents are often included in these behavioral plans.

Family-Based Treatment in More Detail

Because many eating disorders often begin during childhood and adolescence, working with the family was identified as a possible avenue of treatment. Family therapy generally emphasizes the family system as a potential solution for the dilemmas of the eating disorder in young people. Although some important differences have been found between early attempts to involve parents in the treatment of adolescents with eating disorders and more recent work, the groundwork has been laid to bring parents directly into the treatment process because parents are seen as most helpful in resolving the eating disorder in their children. Therefore, family therapy for eating disorders has been seen as a valuable treatment since the mid-1970s.

In general family therapy, the therapist focuses on how family members communicate, how they relate to one another, and how they solve problems. The notion is that in families in which a member has an eating disorder, certain predictable problem areas become evident, such as parents allowing a child to function as an authority figure in the family, avoidance of addressing problems in the interest of keeping the peace, and anxiety about allowing an adolescent child to be independent. The focus of this form of family therapy is not on symptoms or symptom management, as in FBT, but instead on these more general family process concerns.

Several noncontrolled trials of family therapy (in which a series of patients receive the same treatment without any comparison treatment) suggest that involving families in treatment is effective at least for younger patients with anorexia nervosa. Child psychiatrist Salvador Minuchin, who spent most of his professional life at the Child Guidance Clinic in Philadelphia, conducted the most important of these early studies. He and his team reported good outcomes (recovery) in more than 85% of their patients in a case series of 53 adolescents with anorexia. All these patients were treated with family therapy. The other seminal research in family therapy was conducted at the Maudsley Hospital in London. Although this early work was not manualized, many of the main interventions used in what has become FBT were identified by this group in a treatment that became colloquially named "the Maudsley Approach."

A main difference of this approach from other family therapies is that it does not assume that there is something "wrong" with families but instead regards families as often the best resource in treatment. Recovery of the teenager can be accelerated by successfully getting the family on board in treatment, helping the therapist resolve the eating disorder symptoms (the starvation), and getting the young person back on track with adolescent development. This group has gone to conduct studies of a version of family treatment called family therapy for anorexia nervosa (FT-AN) and multifamily group therapy for anorexia nervosa (MFT-AN). The studies of MFT-AN appear to demonstrate some benefits over FT-AN, but there remains much work to be done to assess whether the approach is truly helpful. FT-AN resembles FBT, but no randomized studies have examined it compared to family treatments other than MFT-AN.

Ten randomized clinical trials have examined manualized FBT—a systematic version of the approach by the clinician–researchers at the Maudsley Hospital. These studies produced a number of important findings. First, patients and their families did not drop out of treatment when using FBT. The adolescents in these studies were typical of the type of teens who come for treatment for anorexia nervosa. Most important, FBT was as good as or better than any of the treatments that it has been compared to so far. The first study to use manualized FBT compared a short 6-month course of FBT to a longer course lasting 1 year. There were no differences overall, suggesting that FBT could be effective in a short time. However, for families where there was a single parent or divorced parents, longer treatment was better. Adolescents who had very high levels of obsessive features about eating also did better with longer treatment. Another study compared FBT to AFT and found that it led to faster weight gain, decreased hospitalization use, and higher recovery rates by a margin of two to one. Several studies have followed the adolescents who were treated with FBT and found that most continued to do well several years after treatment. One multisite study compared FBT to systemic family therapy and identified no differences in clinical outcomes between the two treatments, but FBT was more efficient in promoting weight restoration, used less hospitalization during treatment, and was more acceptable to parents than systemic family therapy. Further study of systemic family therapy is likely warranted, as these results are promising for this approach.

Versions of FBT where parents are seen without their child have produced results similar to those that involve the entire family and may be useful for families that struggle with not being critical of one another. More recently a preliminary study of the guided self-help version of FBT (GSH-FBT) found it to be as helpful and used much less therapist time, so it was more cost-effective. Further study of GSH-FBT is underway to see if this finding holds up with a larger sample. Importantly, recent studies of FBT suggest it is as effective when delivered by video as in person, which could allow more families to access treatment. Finally, a study confirmed that early response to FBT is associated with weight gain of about 5 pounds (2.4 kilograms) by the beginning of the fourth session. Early response is highly predictive of outcome over time. For those who do not respond early and whose parents initially feel very ineffective in helping them, adding intensive parent coaching (IPC) helps them recover. IPC involves helping parents understand better why they are being ineffective and includes an additional in vivo meal.

Individual Psychodynamic Psychotherapy in More Detail

As mentioned in Chapter 2, a variety of individual psychotherapies are available, but one kind of therapy your child with anorexia nervosa, bulimia nervosa, or binge-eating disorder is most likely to receive at this time is psychodynamic therapy. This means the treatment will focus more on "underlying issues" than on weight and shape concerns and how to restore healthy body weight. This form of treatment addresses the perceived psychological problems that may cause eating disorders. Specifically, adolescents with eating disorders are believed to be immature and highly anxious about a variety of adolescent issues, including assuming independent roles as adults in a responsible manner. Therapy using this model focuses on the symptoms of disordered eating only insofar as they represent an ineffective and dangerous strategy that keeps the adolescent from addressing her real concerns and issues. Psychodynamic therapy for eating disorders is often relatively unstructured in nature and is not time limited, with treatment goals that are not necessarily very specific. Nevertheless, there is some evidence to support this treatment. In two trials, Arthur Crisp and his colleagues at St. George's Hospital in London reported substantial improvements in their patient groups (these included both adolescents and adults) in terms of both medical/nutritional recovery and psychological improvement, using individual therapy approaches. Many colleagues who practice this approach are mindful of the fact that it may be difficult to do intensive psychotherapy early in treatment when someone is very starved, and consequently, they will adapt their treatments to reflect this reality.

An exception to these general comments about the nonspecificity of individual psychodynamic therapy is the approach developed by Arthur Robin and colleagues at Wayne State University in Detroit, originally called ego-oriented individual therapy and now called AFT for anorexia. Derived from the psychodynamic tradition, AFT aims at maturational issues associated with puberty and adolescence. AFT devised for anorexia nervosa posits that individuals with anorexia nervosa are immature and unaware of their emotions, particularly strong emotions such as anger and depression. These adolescents do not want to face such problems, so they turn to controlling food and weight as a way to keep their feelings and conflicts from surfacing. Thus, according to these theories, eating disorders disrupt normal psychological and physical maturity during adolescence. To develop better ability to manage the challenges of adolescence, they must first learn to identify, define, and tolerate their emotions. In addition, a primary goal of AFT is to foster the adolescent's separation and individuation from the family.

Robin and colleagues used AFT in a randomized clinical trial comparing it with family therapy. The comparison revealed that at the end of treatment family therapy resulted in greater improvements, but at 1-year follow-up there were no significant differences between the two approaches in how patients did. About two-thirds of the adolescents did better overall. This study suggests that AFT is effective, though slower in achieving results than family therapy. What may distinguish AFT from other psychodynamic therapies is the degree to which parents are involved in the treatment, though they specifically did not directly manage eating or other compensatory behaviors like binge eating or purging. As noted earlier, the relatively large randomized clinical trial comparing AFT and FBT found that although overall FBT was more effective, for some that were not as severely ill with obsessions, cognitions, and purging, AFT did almost as well as FBT. For these reasons, AFT is a reasonable evidence-based alternative to FBT when families do not want to do FBT.

Cognitive-Behavioral Therapy for Eating Disorders in Youth in More Detail

The cognitive-behavioral model of bulimia nervosa assumes that the main factors involved in the maintenance of the disorder are problematic *attitudes* toward body shape and weight. Such attitudes lead to an overvaluation of thinness, to dissatisfaction with the body, and to attempts to control shape and weight through excessive dieting. This restrictive pattern of eating then results in both psychological and physiological deprivation, which are often associated with a depressed mood. As a result of the dietary restriction, hunger is increased, leading to an enhanced probability of binge eating, particularly in the presence of depressed mood. Because binge eating raises concerns about gaining weight, it is eventually followed by purging in an attempt to compensate for calories consumed during the binge-eating episode. Based on this model, treatment for bulimia nervosa using CBT focuses first on helping to change eating patterns to make them more normal (that is, three meals and snacks without long periods of fasting between them) so that the urge to binge eat (and therefore purge as well) is decreased. Next, the treatment focuses on the effect of overvaluation of shape and weight on self-esteem and other related thoughts that support an excessive preoccupation with these matters and lead to disordered eating behaviors. Finally, the treatment focuses on what might be expected to lead to a return of eating problems in the future and helps determine what might be done to prevent a relapse.

Different groups of investigators in several countries have completed a number of randomized controlled trials of CBT for bulimia nervosa in adults. Almost all these studies have demonstrated that CBT is the treatment of choice for adults with bulimia nervosa. More specifically, these studies have shown that CBT produces a mean reduction in binge eating and purging of about 70% and a mean abstinence rate from these symptoms approaching 50%. Dietary restraint is also lessened significantly, and the disturbed attitudes toward body weight and shape are greatly reduced. Several studies have shown good maintenance of change at follow-up, ranging from 6 months to 6 years.

CBT is also an effective treatment for adults with binge-eating disorder. The treatment model is similar to that developed for bulimia nervosa except that there is no focus on purging, as it is not present in those with this disorder. Instead the main focus is managing negative attitudes toward the body, self, food, and weight. There is some research data supporting that CBT may be helpful for youth with binge-eating disorder, but further systematic data are needed.

CBT has also been studied for children, adolescents, and adults with ARFID. Again, the general model is similar to that developed for bulimia nervosa in adults, but for younger children parental behavioral management strategies similar to FBT are incorporated. Thus far, CBT has led to improvements in the symptoms of ARFID, but no randomized treatment comparisons have yet been conducted, so it is unknown how it compares to other approaches.

Interpersonal Psychotherapy for Bulimia Nervosa and Binge-Eating Disorder

Another effective treatment for adults with bulimia nervosa is IPT. IPT was initially developed as a brief treatment for depression and anxiety problems in adults. It is based on the idea that emotional problems are best conceived of as a result of interpersonal problems, particularly current ones. Treatment for bulimia nervosa using IPT also focuses on the interpersonal context within which the eating disorder developed and is maintained, with the aim of helping the patient make specific changes in identified interpersonal problem areas. So, in direct distinction from CBT, the focus is not on changing behaviors or cognitions related directly to bulimia. In fact, little attention is paid to eating habits or attitudes toward weight and shape. Several studies now provide empirical support for the use of IPT to treat bulimia nervosa, though none have shown it to be superior to CBT. IPT can probably be helpful to adolescents with bulimia nervosa, but in order to be optimally effective with young people it may require modifications to include a greater role for parents. When parents are included in treatment, they can provide support and encouragement as well as direct assistance in helping to change bulimic behaviors and attitudes.

Nutritional Counseling

Another approach commonly used for treating eating disorders is nutritional counseling. Nutritionists have long played a role in this treatment, on the assumption that their expertise in diets and health can help patients reevaluate their choices along more reasonable guidelines. Usual nutritional counseling consists of providing meal plans, caloric recommendations, discussion of alternative food choices to meet nutritional requirements, and support for continued progress in making healthier food choices. To date, however, the few studies that have examined this treatment have been conducted with adult patients and have found that other psychological treatments (family therapy and individual therapy) are superior to nutritional counseling. However, it may be helpful at times to consult with a nutritionist for guidance on specific nutritional requirements or difficulties.

In summary, the research literature suggests that two forms of outpatient psychotherapy may be effective for anorexia nervosa: FBT and AFT. Up to this point, FBT has received greater attention and has more evidence to support it. However, the tradition of psychodynamic psychotherapy lends additional credibility to AFT. For bulimia nervosa, FBT appears to be the best and most efficient approach, but CBT is also a reasonable alternative for youth with this disorder. CBT likely needs to include parents in some capacity to maximize effectiveness when used with young people. As noted, CBT is effective for binge-eating disorders in adults and likely useful for older adolescents. Furthermore, CBT and FBT are both good candidates for treating youth with ARFID. IPT is also a likely effective treatment for adults with bulimia nervosa, and it has been shown to be helpful for teenagers with depression, so it may be a reasonable option, especially if interpersonal factors are clearly identified as problematic. Again, though, family involvement is usually crucial to work with adolescents in IPT. The role of nutritional counseling remains uncertain from a research perspective, though this treatment alone appears to be inadequate for most patients. Integrated into other psychological interventions, however, nutritional counseling may still have a role.

Psychiatric Medications

In addition to psychological outpatient treatments, a variety of medications have been studied to see if they are of benefit for eating disorders. Although psychotropic medications—medications that are exclusively developed for the treatment of psychiatric illnesses—can be helpful for some, it's important to appreciate how little we know about the efficacy of medications in the treatment of eating disorders.

Antidepressant and antianxiety medications have been examined in adults with anorexia nervosa and found to be of limited help, especially during periods when these patients were acutely medically compromised. Many earlier, smaller studies have demonstrated few significant improvements in patients as a result of psychopharmacological intervention. A recent, larger randomized clinical trial of adults with anorexia nervosa found that adding an atypical antipsychotic improved weight gain, on average; however, it should be noted that the amount of weight gain was not particularly large. The role of medications in adolescents with anorexia nervosa has received little attention, but the studies conducted have not demonstrated systematic benefit for any of the medications examined, including antidepressants, anxiolytics, appetite stimulants, and antipsychotics. While these medications may be used to manage short-term behavioral or emotional reactivity, they appear to do little to help with the main symptoms of anorexia nervosa, and parents are advised not to place too much hope in them as a solution. Overall, the conclusion you should draw from this limited work is that the benefits of medication in the treatment of anorexia nervosa remain at best uncertain. In fact, most clinicians will agree that *the best medicine for anorexia remains food at a dose of three meals and three snacks per day!*

Yet, please keep in mind that several other psychiatric illnesses, such as depression and anxiety, may co-occur with anorexia nervosa, as discussed in Chapter 4. If your child has such a co-occurring disorder, she may very well benefit from a course of antidepressant or antianxiety medication, as long as the medication is prescribed for the depression or the anxiety. In addition, there are a host of medical complications for anorexia nervosa, as we have elaborated on earlier,

Understand Your Options

and many patients benefit from several nonpsychotropic medications that your pediatrician can prescribe to deal with abdominal discomfort or any other medical complication associated with your child's illness. However, it should also be noted that although many young people appear to meet the criteria for many psychiatric disorders (for example, anxiety disorder, depression, obsessive–compulsive disorder, autism spectrum disorder), when they are acutely ill and malnourished, most "recover" from these other disorders when anorexia nervosa is effectively treated. This suggests that these were not really "separate" disorders, but really a part of the overall clinical picture of anorexia nervosa.

In contrast to these discouraging findings about the help medications might offer for anorexia, most studies show convincing evidence that supports the use of antidepressant medications for adults with bulimia nervosa and binge-eating disorder. Researchers were prompted to pursue the use of these medications precisely because so many patients with bulimia nervosa also prove to be suffering from depression when they consult their doctors. Inasmuch as antidepressant medications are helpful in depression, they may also be helpful in bulimia nervosa and binge-eating disorder. These observations led to a series of double-blind, placebo-controlled trials of antidepressants among adult patients with bulimia nervosa and binge-eating disorder. In such a trial, neither the researchers nor the study participants know who is taking the medication under investigation or the placebo (sugar pill). Most classes of antidepressant medications have been tested in these studies, including the tricyclics, monoamine oxidase inhibitors (MAOIs), selective serotonin reuptake inhibitors (SSRIs), and atypical antidepressants such as bupropion and trazodone. In almost all these studies, both tricyclics and fluoxetine (the SSRI most commonly known by the trade name Prozac) have proven to be better than the placebo in terms of the reduction in binge frequency. Generally, depression and preoccupation with shape and weight also show greater improvement with medication as opposed to placebo pills. However, overall response to medication treatment alone for bulimia nervosa is less than for psychological treatment alone.

Cognitive-Behavioral Therapy and Medications in Combination

Several controlled studies have looked at medication *and* psychotherapy treatments for bulimia in adults. These studies evaluated the relative (medication versus psychotherapy) as well as the combined (medication plus psychotherapy) effectiveness of CBT and antidepressant drug treatment. These studies indicate that (1) CBT is superior to medication alone, (2) combining CBT with medication is significantly more effective than medication alone, and (3) combining CBT and medication provides only modest incremental benefits over CBT alone. The result is that patients who receive CBT versus medication are often less likely to drop out of treatment. A recent meta-analysis (combining data from several studies to increase statistical significance) of psychosocial and pharmacological treatment studies for adult bulimia confirmed CBT as the treatment of choice. Taken together, these outcomes mean that *just* receiving antidepressant medication is seldom sufficient for bulimia. So when medications are used, other psychological treatments (for example, CBT) should almost always be included. Another finding that favors CBT is that psychotherapies are usually more acceptable to patients as compared with medication. The benefits of medication treatment for binge-eating disorder are not as clear. Medications alone appear to be helpful for many. Studies of medication treatments for ARFID do not yet exist. However, antidepressants are sometimes used to decrease anxiety about eating and swallowing as well as stimulate appetite.

In summary, recent studies of treatment for adults with bulimia and binge-eating disorder have demonstrated that CBT and antidepressant medications (especially SSRIs such as Prozac) are potentially effective treatments. No treatment study that exclusively involves adolescents with bulimia nervosa or binge-eating disorder has been published, however. Until adolescents are studied, whether treatments that have shown to be helpful for adults can be applied to adolescents will remain speculative. As a parent, you might want to make sure that your doctor appreciates this fact and exercises the necessary caution when prescribing medications. Even if these treatments can be applied to adolescents, we do not know whether they are as effective for adolescents as for adults. You should therefore carefully question your doctor in terms of how she might apply these findings gathered from adults with bulimia to your adolescent.

INTENSIVE TREATMENTS

Unfortunately, a significant minority of those with anorexia nervosa, and many with bulimia nervosa, who are critically ill may require a period of inpatient treatment. Inpatient, day-patient, and residential treatments all have one thing in common: Your child receives treatment at a health care facility, either full time or for a large portion of each day. This usually means that you will not be involved in the day-to-day management of your child's eating problems, although the treatment team may work with you to varying degrees, depending on the therapeutic approach of the facility. In this section, we discuss the scientific support available suggesting that intensive treatments such as inpatient hospital programs are helpful for eating disorders.

Many parents we've counseled have expressed confusion about the differences between inpatient, day-patient, and residential treatments. Inpatient treatment is usually indicated when someone is in urgent need of weight restoration or has other acute medical problems associated with an eating disorder. Once these problems are addressed, many patients are transferred to a day-patient program. Here the patient is further encouraged to gain weight and eliminate other disordered eating behaviors but gets to go home every evening and weekend. Finally, residential treatment looks a lot like an inpatient program but usually serves the purpose of accommodating those patients who may have "failed" other treatments and require quite a lengthy stay (up to several months) to help them get back on track. In essence, though, there are perhaps more similarities than differences between these three intensive treatment approaches.

All three forms of intensive treatment attempt to first restore weight and stop or significantly decrease binge eating and purging, if these are concerns. Second, the programs aim to help the patients learn to manage continuing health on their own and assist the patients through a variety of forms of psychotherapy to reach an improved understanding of why they developed an eating disorder or are maintaining one. All the while, the patients are supported and encouraged through psychotherapeutic meetings in a group format and, often, in family therapy settings as well.

However, in addition to providing psychological insight-oriented therapies, many such programs, it's fair to say, follow a behavioral approach. What this means (again, whether in an inpatient, day-patient, or residential setting) is that a primary focus of day-to-day activity will be on eating and disordered eating behaviors. In practice, this means that for those who are severely underweight, independence will initially be restricted so as to conserve energy; as they gain weight, they will also be released from the restriction of bed rest or may start participating in a supervised but limited exercise program. For those with unremitting binge-eating or purging or overexercising behaviors, close observation by professional staff is designed to prevent those behaviors, with the idea that disrupting the chronic practice of these behaviors will help reduce their recurrence. Overall, these prohibitions and observations by professional staff are decreased as the patient demonstrates improvement. The idea is that the patient gains greater freedom, in terms of both independence and food decisions, as she returns to normal weight and eating behaviors. These activities take place in all three of these treatment settings, with the difference often being the length of stay and the number of hours spent in the treatment setting from day to day, as well as the extent to which and the speed at which independence is encouraged and permitted.

Several investigators have published reports on the effectiveness of hospitalization in the treatment of anorexia nervosa, but there are no comparable studies for bulimia nervosa. In most cases, specialist units are quite successful at refeeding patients and restoring a healthy body weight. For example, one study found overall clinical improvement in the 16 participating patients after an average of 3 months of inpatient treatment using a behavioral approach, whereby the patient gains more freedom/rewards as weight increases. Also using a behavioral approach, another researcher found that 70% of patients showed continued improvement at 3-year follow-up when treated for a period of 6 months as inpatients. However, a large study conducted in the United Kingdom of 167 adolescents with anorexia nervosa who were randomly treated with a 16-week hospital stay or two forms of outpatient therapy found no differences in outcomes between the groups, except that the cost of treatment was much greater in those who were treated in the hospital. This means that for most adolescents with anorexia nervosa, an inpatient treatment program is not more helpful than outpatient treatment. This does not mean hospital treatment is not needed for some adolescents with anorexia nervosa. That is, those who are medically unstable and those who struggle to make weight gains in outpatient treatment should be in the hospital. However, the study strongly suggests that inpatient treatment is not necessarily the first step parents should consider in treating their child. In another recent study, adolescents with anorexia nervosa were randomized to receive a short medical hospitalization for stabilization of low heart rates and low blood pressure or a longer medical hospitalization aimed at weight restoration. At discharge, all participants received FBT. At the end of 1 year of treatment and 1 year of follow-up, there were no differences in clinical outcomes, rates of readmission to hospital, or use of other therapies between the two groups. This meant that a short medical hospitalization followed by FBT is as effective clinically as restoring adolescents to near normal weight before starting FBT. However, overall, the costs of treatment were much lower for the group that received the shorter hospital treatment.

These studies together indicate that inpatient treatment is likely to result in short-term clinical improvement, but the longer-term benefits are uncertain. It's important to keep in mind, though, that what happens in study settings is often very different from what happens in reality. For instance, a study protocol may allow for relatively lengthy treatment stays, whereas in practice you may find that your insurance company will pay for only a few weeks of treatment.

One of the discouraging aspects of inpatient treatment is that within a few short weeks of discharge many patients promptly lose the weight they painstakingly gained, even when they have had months of intensive treatment. For instance, one researcher who reviewed inpatient treatments reported that at least 40% of hospitalized patients are readmitted at least once. Furthermore, this report indicated that patients with eating disorders spent *more* time in the hospital with each succeeding admission than any other patient group with non-organic disorders. In other words, many patients, especially those with anorexia, seem to spend an inordinate amount of their young lives in hospitals. We've pointed out that for many patients inpatient stays are, unfortunately, necessary. Several recent studies have found that adolescents who are treated with FBT typically require fewer admissions and have shorter stays than those who receive other therapies. To us this finding suggests that for adolescents, in particular, it is likely best to try to help them at home, with their family and friends available to support them.

WHAT CONCLUSIONS SHOULD YOU DRAW ABOUT THE TREATMENTS AVAILABLE FOR EATING DISORDERS?

The results from the empirical data so far available about all the treatments reviewed in this chapter fall within the modest-to-moderate range, and treatment studies to date are few. Still, several clear guidelines have emerged from these studies, as well as from our own experience with patients.

First, it's of paramount importance that you act early when your child shows signs of an eating disorder. Please don't hesitate or worry that you'll be seen as overreacting or interfering. Detecting and treating any illness in its early stages is invariably more favorable than waiting for the symptoms to set in and become more intractable.

Second, your involvement, especially in outpatient treatments, should be the rule and not the exception. Although you may feel ill-equipped to tackle an illness as severe as an eating disorder, this concern is usually unfounded. Eating disorders are complex illnesses, and successful treatment often requires the dedicated efforts of a team of professionals (psychologists, psychiatrists, pediatricians, and nutritionists). Each of these professionals will help with your adolescent's treatment program, and each will address an important part of the problem. You should be able to count on the expertise of these professionals, but they should also recognize the important contribution you can make. No matter how your child came to have an eating disorder, as a parent you know your child best and you spend more time with your son or daughter than do any of the professionals on the treatment team. You not only have a lot to offer, your participation is critical because your teenager will be under your supervision more than anyone else's.

Third, early and careful attention to medical problems associated with eating disorders is critical. Too often, energetic attempts at addressing the causes of the illness are pursued prior to taking care of the life-threatening symptoms of an eating disorder. If your parental instinct tells you your child is in trouble, but the professional you consult wants to explore why your daughter won't eat or why your son is throwing up his dinner every night, insist on immediate attention to the urgent problem at hand: restoring your child's health. If you and the practitioner can't agree on that course of action, you need to find another expert (see Chapter 10). Most clinicians will, of course, have your teenager's best interests at heart and should be willing to work with you in returning your child to health. In the next two chapters, we discuss just how you can make sure that you're productively involved in your child's treatment, regardless of the specific treatment received.

FOR MORE INFORMATION

Agras, W. S., J. Lock, H. Brandt, et al., Comparison of 2 Family Therapies for Adolescent Anorexia Nervosa: A Randomized Trial, *JAMA Psychiatry*, 71(11), 1279–1286.

Andersen, A., W. Bowers, and K. Evans, Inpatient Treatment of Anorexia Nervosa, in D. M. Garner and P. E. Garfinkel, Editors, *Handbook of Treatment for Eating Disorders, Second Edition*, 1997. New York: Guilford Press, pp. 327–353.

Couturier, J., and J. Lock, Review of Medication Use for Children and Adolescents with Eating Disorders, *Journal of the Canadian Academy of Child and Adolescent Psychiatry*, 2007, 16, 173–176.

Dalle Grave, R., M. Conti, M. Sartirana, et al., Enhanced Cognitive Behavioral Therapy for Adolescents with Eating Disorders: A Systematic Review of Current Status and Future Perspectives, *International Journal of Eating Disorders and Obesity*, 2021, *3*, 1–11.

Datta, N., B. Matheson, K. Citron, et al., Evidence-Based Update on Psychosocial Interventions for Eating Disorders in Children and Adolescents, *Journal of Clinical Child and Adolescent Psychology*, 2023, *52*(2), 159–170.

Gowers, S. G., A. Clark, C. Roberts, et al., Clinical Effectiveness of Treatments for Anorexia Nervosa in Adolescents: Randomised Controlled Trial, *British Journal of Psychiatry*, 2007, *191*, 427–435.

Hagman, J., J. Gralla, E. Sigel, et al., A Double-Blind, Placebo-Controlled Study of Risperidone for the Treatment of Adolescents and Young Adults with Anorexia Nervosa: A Pilot Study, *American Journal of Child and Adolescent Psychiatry*, 2011, *50*, 915–924.

Le Grange, D., R. Crosby, P. Rathouz, et al., A Randomized Controlled Comparison of Family-Based Treatment and Supportive Psychotherapy for Adolescent Bulimia Nervosa, *Archives of General Psychiatry*, 2007, *64*, 1049–1056.

Le Grange, D., S. Eckhardt, R. Dalle Grave, et al., Enhanced Cognitive-Behavior Therapy and Family-Based Treatment for Adolescents with an Eating Disorder: A Non-randomized Effectiveness Trial, *Psychological Medicine*, 2020, *52*(13), 1–11.

Le Grange, D., E. Hughes, A. Court, et al., Randomized Clinical Trial of Parent Focused Therapy and Family-Based Treatment for Adolescent Anorexia Nervosa, *Journal of the American Academy of Child and Adolescent Psychiatry*, 2016, *55*(8), 683–692.

Le Grange, D., J. Lock, W. Agras, et al., Randomized Clinical Trial of Family-Based Treatment and Cognitive-Behavioral Therapy for Adolescent Bulimia Nervosa, *Journal of the American Academy of Child and Adolescent Psychiatry*, 2015, *54*(11), 886–894.

Lock, J., Adjusting Cognitive Behavioral Therapy for Adolescent Bulimia Nervosa: Results of a Case Series, *American Journal of Psychotherapy*, 2005, *59*, 267–281.

Lock, J., W. S. Agras, S. Bryson, et al., A Comparison of Short- and Long-Term Family Therapy for Adolescent Anorexia Nervosa, *Journal of the American Academy of Child and Adolescent Psychiatry*, 2005, *44*, 632–639.

Lock, J., J. Couturier, B. Matheson, et al., Feasibility of Conducting a Randomized Clinical Trial Comparing Family-Based Treatment via Teleconferencing and Online Guided Self-Help Family-Based Treatment for Adolescent Anorexia Nervosa, *International Journal of Eating Disorders,* 2021, *54*(11), 1998–2008.

Lock, J., D. Le Grange, W. S. Agras, et al., A Randomized Clinical Trial Comparing Family-Based Treatment to Adolescent Focused Individual Therapy for Adolescents with Anorexia Nervosa, *Archives of General Psychiatry,* 2010, *67,* 1025–1032.

Lock, J., D. Le Grange, C. Bohon, et al., Who Responds to an Adaptive Treatment for Adolescents with Anorexia Nervosa? Outcomes from a Randomized Clinical Trial, *Journal of the American Academy of Child and Adolescent Psychiatry,* 2024, *63*(6), 605–614.

Lock, J., S. Sadeh-Sharvit, and A. L'Insalata, Feasibility of Conducting a Randomized Clinical Trial Using Family-Based Treatment for Avoidant/Restrictive Food Intake Disorder, *International Journal of Eating Disorders,* 2019, *52,* 746–751.

Madden, S., J. Miskovic-Wheatley, A. Wallis, et al., A Randomized Controlled Trial of Inpatient Hospitalization for Anorexia Nervosa in Medically Unstable Adolescents, *Psychological Medicine,* 2014, *44,* 1053–1064.

PART III

MAKING TREATMENT WORK

How to Solve Everyday Problems to Help Your Child Recover

CHAPTER 7

Taking Charge of Change

How to Apply Family-Based Treatment to Help with Eating Disorders

"We've tried everything. We tried letting her decide. We tried to force her to eat. We threatened her. We've punished her. Nothing works."

This is what we typically hear from parents who have just been told they will be taking direct responsibility for getting their child to return to normal eating patterns. If you're involved in a form of treatment that asks you to take charge of normalizing eating behavior for your adolescent—such as FBT—you may initially be perplexed and doubtful and perhaps even frustrated by the request. Parents tell us they don't know *how* to get their son or daughter to eat—either enough or regularly. Naturally, this is a source of exasperation and increasing frustration for them. It can also feel as if the situation is creating a great rift between the parents and the child who doesn't want to eat or who wants to purge. Many parents end up feeling as if they're fighting not just this illness but the child they're trying desperately to help as well.

In this chapter and the next, we discuss the range of ways you can become practically involved in helping your adolescent with various problems related to eating disorders. This chapter focuses on the FBT approach, which informs much of this book's basic premise, wherein you are asked to be *directly responsible* for changing eating-related behaviors at home. If your child is receiving a different kind of treatment that does not ask you to take this responsibility—or even discourages it—you can and should still be involved in your child's return to health; you'll find suggestions on how to do so within the other forms of therapy used for eating disorders (described in Chapter 6) in Chapter 8.

Whether the abnormal eating pattern is related to anorexia nervosa, bulimia nervosa, binge eating, or avoidant/restrictive food intake disorder (ARFID), you will be surprised by how successful you can be in helping your child without resorting to threats, punishments, or berating. The leverage you have as parents that no one else has is your love and commitment to your child. This is powerful leverage.

You are naturally anxious about your child's health and welfare, and this may make you unsure about what to do. A certain degree of anxiety is a good thing—it helps propel you to action—but too much anxiety can overwhelm and immobilize you. There is no denying that finding ways to help your child eat normally is challenging. You may try things that don't work well. For example, some parents try to "sneak" butter or other fat into foods. This sounds like a good idea from a nutritional perspective, but it usually leads to the child's distrusting you. We have found it better to be very clear and specific about expectations as well as very direct in stating them. This is just one example of the principles we can offer to guide you in coming up with your own ways to help your teenager begin to eat healthily again. Throughout this chapter our goal will be to help you gain confidence in your ability to handle this problem, as you have handled so many other dilemmas of parenthood, thereby alleviating anxiety.

Excessive anxiety only makes parents hesitant, which leads to another problem. Your lack of confidence and your uncertainty will often be perceived as a lack of resolve. This encourages your child to resist you even more because of the hold the eating disorder has on her. As we said in Chapter 1, don't hesitate. Act now.

Taking Charge of Change

A FEW FUNDAMENTAL PRINCIPLES

As with many behavioral problems in children, some fundamental guidelines will apply here. First, come up with an approach to helping your child eat normally that you can carry out. It's not much help to say you will eat all meals with your son if you're working all day and can't possibly be there. Second, be reasonable in your expectations of both yourself and your child for making behavior changes. Changing behaviors will take some time; prepare to be patient. Third, use strategies that respect your child, but guard against succumbing to pressures to let up on your expectations. This means remembering that your child has an illness and is not fully in control of his thinking and actions. In addition, it means being sympathetic and caring rather than critical and punishing. Fourth, make sure you have support, both from other family members and friends and from professionals, because this is going to be difficult at times. If the challenge were not difficult, this kind of action on your part would not be warranted to begin with. Finally, make sure you don't give up too soon. Sometimes early success leads to lowering your guard too soon, allowing the eating problem to resurface.

When you're involved in FBT, the following specific principles will apply:

1. Work with experts who know how to help you.
2. Work together as a family.
3. Don't blame your child or yourself for the problems you're having. Blame the illness.
4. Focus on the problem before you.
5. Don't debate with your child about eating- or weight-related concerns.
6. Know when to begin backing off.
7. Take care of yourself. You are your child's best hope.

The rest of this chapter is dedicated to examining each of these principles in turn. To illustrate, throughout the chapter we describe the experiences of many of the families we've helped treat, in addition to following 15-year-old Cindy, as she and her family take up the challenge of fighting anorexia nervosa together.

> Cindy was a very focused teenager. Her father, Jorge, was an accountant, and her mother, Susan, was a real estate agent. She also had a 17-year-old brother, Todd, who attended the same high school. Cindy had always been an excellent student, though she was also somewhat shy socially. She began dieting when she was a freshman because she felt she could "improve" herself if she was more fit and healthy. As she lost weight, some girlfriends commented that she looked "really good," and this made Cindy feel more accepted and liked. However, in a few months Cindy's parents became alarmed at her weight loss. She now weighed 80 pounds at a height of 5 feet even. When her parents took her to her pediatrician, she referred Cindy and her parents to a family therapist, who used family treatment that asked Jorge and Susan to take initial responsibility for refeeding Cindy.

WORK WITH EXPERTS WHO KNOW HOW TO HELP YOU

We discussed the importance of expert evaluation and treatment in Chapter 1. This is particularly important if you're going to be in charge of directly changing eating-disordered behaviors in your home. By now you know that understanding eating disorders is not a simple matter. So, the more experience your expert has had in helping families with these problems, the deeper his understanding of the complexities of these disorders will be. And the deeper the expert's understanding, the more assistance you're likely to receive in refining your own understanding of why you may be having difficulty changing your child's eating-related behavior.

Although we strongly believe you have the skills to help your son or daughter with an eating disorder, applying those skills effectively usually requires help. An expert consults with you about what you're doing and advises you to examine what works and doesn't work. An expert with a great deal of experience can offer advice on how to

Taking Charge of Change

improve your current efforts or what to consider when you feel you've hit a brick wall.

At the same time, an expert can help you better understand your child's thinking. This is important, because at first it will appear to your child that the therapist is "on your side" and against her. By helping you better understand the illness, the therapist demonstrates an understanding of your child's experience to the child, inspiring greater trust and cooperation with treatment over time.

The expert therapist will also understand that every family is different and has its own style of self-management and problem solving. An experienced therapist will be able to identify the common threads that tie together all families struggling with eating disorders without imposing one-size-fits-all recommendations. The details regarding a therapist's former patients and the examples we offer in this chapter won't necessarily be completely transferable to your own family. That's where your therapist comes in. The therapist is there to help you make these principles pertinent and particular to your family.

WORK TOGETHER AS A FAMILY

In our experience, parents have indeed tried many things in their efforts to help their son or daughter change the self-destructive eating patterns of anorexia, bulimia, and ARFID; usually, however, they haven't tried any tactic consistently, confidently, and with clear commitment from both parents (see Chapter 9).

> After their first family therapy meeting, Jorge and Susan, parents of Cindy, felt overwhelmed and bewildered. The therapist had told them to find a way to make Cindy eat. Jorge sat down with Cindy and asked her what she would eat. Cindy said she would eat her rice and steamed vegetables. Susan said she wanted her to eat a piece of chicken. Cindy refused. Susan told her she must eat it. This led to a shouting match that ended when Cindy left the table without eating anything.
>
> When Cindy's therapist met with the family next, she listened carefully to what had happened. First, she asked the parents if the two of them agreed that Cindy needed to eat the

chicken as well as the rice and vegetables. They agreed about that. However, Jorge said he couldn't stand all the yelling that went on and was happy to see Cindy eat anything. It was apparent to the therapist that although Jorge and Susan agreed about what should be done, they did not have the same threshold for what that meant. The therapist explained that it was just this kind of "gap" in the plan that allowed the eating disorder to slip through and reduce their effectiveness. The therapist suggested that Susan and Jorge work together to refine their plan to include what the threshold for eating enough would be and what they would do to enforce it.

The next day Jorge and Susan went out for coffee. They agreed that Cindy had to eat chicken in addition to rice and vegetables. They also agreed that she would need to eat one chicken breast, but they would allow her to choose how it should be prepared. They, not she, would prepare it, however.

What Jorge and Susan did was take a *first step* toward identifying a solution to breaking the hold anorexia had on Cindy. There would be many more steps in their struggle. There are many ways that parents can *seem* to be working together, but when push comes to shove, they are not. Often they can even be working at cross-purposes. This scenario is so common we've devoted an entire chapter to it (Chapter 9). For now, though, it's important to realize how critical it is that you and your child's other parent or any other adult in the household present a united front in trying to reestablish normal eating behavior.

Dinah's mother diligently made her eat her meals, but her father, who believed that allowing Dinah to exercise would help motivate her to eat, took her running or to the gym most nights, effectively undermining any weight gain as she used up more calories with this exercise than she took in.

Neither of Dinah's parents was "wrong," but because they didn't connect the two parts of the plan, they were not successful in working together.

Haddiyah's mother resented doing any direct refeeding and was angry about it, though she professed to her husband that she was behind the effort. Haddiyah's mother would "be around" during mealtimes but did not really pay attention to whether Haddiyah was actually eating. Haddiyah knew this and easily slipped most of her food into the trash. Thus, it appeared to everyone that Haddiyah's lack of progress was inexplicable.

Again, neither of Haddiyah's parents was wrong. They just hadn't really agreed to the treatment approach. It turned out that Haddiyah's mother felt that her husband had bullied her into this kind of treatment and she had not wished to confront him directly.

Tammy's father had abandoned the family when she was just a baby. There was no other extended family nearby either, so Tammy and her mother were very close. In the case of Tammy's mother, the conflict was with herself. On the one hand, she felt she had to keep her daughter from purging every day, but on the other, she felt so terrible about "watching and controlling" her teenage daughter that she found herself giving in and "ignoring" the obvious signs that Tammy was purging.

Tammy's mother's mixed impulses are very understandable. As we've discussed, the person with an eating disorder often demonstrates perfectly normal thinking in most settings—except where food and weight are concerned. Parents have described mealtimes as similar to watching a "fog" roll over their child's personality and thinking. The teenager appears perfectly normal, but when expected to consume food the parents have designated as appropriate, anger, resentment, and bizarre behaviors emerge. It's very confusing to see your child thinking and acting rationally and then becoming irrational, highly emotional, or withdrawn at mealtime. This confusion may lead to uncertainty and ambivalence about your efforts to refeed your child or prevent binge eating and purging. Like Tammy's mother, you may end up hesitant to do what you need to do. Unfortunately, hesitancy leaves room for eating-disordered thinking to slip through and establish a firmer foothold, as we mentioned earlier. Feelings like those Tammy's mother experienced undermine the success of either taking control and intervening or identifying a different treatment approach (see the next chapter) that might be more consistent with a strong dislike of monitoring the child with the eating disorder.

Don't Exclude Siblings

Your other children are another resource that can help defeat eating disorders. Your own brothers and sisters are the people with whom you will likely have the longest relationships in your life, and this is just as true for your child. Whether or not they show it, siblings are usually affected when one of their own has an eating disorder. They are sometimes aware of the problem before you are. However, they often feel confused, burdened by a mixed obligation to both protect and help their sibling. They can also be angry at the brother or sister with an eating disorder for "causing all these problems" for the family.

In therapy, siblings can help *support* your son or daughter with an eating disorder. First, just by coming to treatment, siblings express their interest and concern. True, at first they may come only because you force them to. However, over time they also benefit from seeing how the family together can be a resource in overcoming a problem, in this case an eating disorder. Younger siblings, ages 5–6, may not understand all that is going on, but the therapist will ask them to do something kind for their sister or brother—such as make a card or do a chore that would ordinarily be done by that sibling. Older siblings may take their brother or sister on an outing to help distract their sibling from feeling miserable about eating and gaining weight or to prevent the sibling from purging. In these ways, and many others, siblings can help make the process of changing problematic eating behaviors in the home easier.

Of course, at times siblings can be unhelpful. Monica and Delphine were twins who had always competed with one another. When Monica began to diet and lost a little weight, Delphine had to take it further. When Delphine developed anorexia, Monica was anything but supportive. She felt she had to be an "even better anorexic" than her sister. In this instance, the continued competition over weight and appearance made it impossible to see the whole family together. Instead, the therapist worked with just the parents and supported each daughter separately while the parents worked to help both of them. Sometimes, brothers can continue to be insulting about weight and ridicule their sisters, though they usually learn to stop.

It's helpful to understand what really lies behind these behaviors. Is it jealousy? Fear or worry? Or is it evidence of an unsalvageable relationship? Your therapist should help you figure out what's behind the behavior and how best to deal with it. In any event, as a parent, you need to act to stop this type of behavior because it will undermine your success.

DON'T BLAME YOUR CHILD OR YOURSELF

It's very difficult not to hold your son or daughter responsible when what you see before you is a child who appears to be obstinately refusing to eat. However, just as we know it's not helpful for you to feel blamed for causing an eating disorder (see Chapter 3), it is clearly also not helpful to blame your child. Remembering that your child has a life-threatening illness that distorts her thinking and experience about her weight and shape can sometimes keep your own thinking clearer about the situation. Still, this is tricky because, of course, your child is there in front of you, and it is her voice saying no and her refusal to adhere to reasonable eating behaviors that is causing the problem. However, she is also clearly miserable and cannot please you or herself in this dilemma. To explain this further, let's return to Cindy's family.

> At their next meeting Cindy's parents complained to the therapist about how much resistance to eating Cindy was putting up and how angry they were at her. The therapist expressed sympathy for the difficulty they were having but, by drawing on the board a Venn diagram of intersecting circles, like the one presented in Chapter 2, reminded them just how differently Cindy was seeing the world through the lens of anorexia nervosa. Then she reminded them that it usually wasn't helpful to blame Cindy for her preoccupation with weight loss. She had an illness that kept her from seeing things the same way others did. The therapist helped the family see how much her anorexia was overshadowing who Cindy really was—she couldn't participate in her school or social life, all her time was spent on worrying about her weight and food, and she had completely lost her sense of

humor. However, the therapist noted that understanding her plight was one thing, but allowing starvation to continue was another. She once again charged them with finding a way to help Cindy eat and fight anorexia. Keeping the illness separate from Cindy was more difficult than it seemed. This was hard on Susan, who still struggled to stop seeing Cindy's eating disorder as "willful," but she said she would try. Jorge also agreed that no matter how hard it was to listen to Cindy's wailing, he would not leave the room.

When dinner time came, Susan and Jorge put the meat they expected Cindy to eat on her plate. Cindy immediately got up and left the table. Calmly, they followed her to her room, brought her dinner with them, and sat next to her on the bed. They gently explained that they knew this was hard on her, they loved her, and they would be there to help her. They sat there for about an hour, and Cindy still refused to eat. Susan began to get angry, and Jorge asked if perhaps she might want to take a break and come back in a minute. Susan thought this was a good idea and did so. Cindy now began to cry and claimed that her dinner was ruined. Jorge explained that he would heat it up and she could eat it. Cindy ate a few bites and climbed into bed. Her parents explained that they would not give up on her and were happy she had eaten some of her dinner with them. Her mother said, "I know how hard it was for you to eat that because anorexia is so powerful. We'll keep trying."

It's important to understand that Cindy and her family were just beginning to work on her anorexia together. At this point, Jorge and Susan had determined that their support and encouragement were the correct response to Cindy's minimal consumption *at this meal*. This did not mean they would allow Cindy to continue to eat too little food to regain weight or even sustain her. An important aspect of fighting an eating disorder is establishing consequences for not eating, as discussed later in this chapter. Setting consequences not only serves as an incentive for the child to eat, but also gives parents another way to respond to not eating other than getting angry and falling prey to the instinct to blame the child for the illness.

It makes perfect sense to hold a healthy teenager responsible for her own behavior. It even makes sense to hold an adolescent with an

Taking Charge of Change 163

eating disorder responsible for behavior that has nothing to do with weight or food. But when it comes to eating and exercise patterns in a child with an eating disorder, it's critical to remember to *separate the illness from the child*. No matter how rational she may sound, no matter how committed she is to her beliefs about eating and weight, your child is not really responsible for what she says and does with regard to food if she has an eating disorder. When you talk to her about these subjects, it's the eating disorder that answers you. And it's the eating disorder you should designate as your foe, never your son or daughter. Many parents naturally have trouble remembering that "no, I won't eat" is not coming from the same source as "no, I don't think I should have to have a curfew." A thorough understanding of the cognitive distortions described in Chapter 5 can, however, help you keep it clear in your mind that you're struggling with an illness rather than with your son or daughter.

> Jackson's father went into a tirade whenever he found evidence that his son was still throwing up. When Jackson's dad got angry, he became critical and hostile, and Jackson felt as though he was being attacked. This led to Jackson's increased efforts to hide the fact that he still hadn't completely stopped purging. This made it hard for his family to see the progress he was making or to see just where he was having continued difficulties. This meant they couldn't help him as effectively.

Anger can throw you off and make it harder for you to know that the illness is the problem and not your child. When helping your child eat, anger will definitely interfere with your success.

Another way you can separate the illness from the child is to keep in mind that your child does not really choose to be ill, even if it appears that way. The child with anorexia nervosa may have little motivation to recover, but it's the illness that is so recalcitrant, rather than your child. Certainly, purging is frustrating because it appears to many people as wasteful and dirty. However, most children who purge their food feel trapped into doing so by their worries and anxieties about weight and have become caught in a chronic cycle that they don't know how to break out of. Keeping these facts in mind may help you contain your anger. It may also help if you try to remember that it's hard for your child to perceive that your anger is directed at the illness and not at her for being willful, ungrateful, difficult, and frustrating.

Still, your anger about having to take on this problem is understandable. You certainly don't deserve this—and neither does your child. To keep your anger from either overwhelming you or being vented on your child, it's important to recognize the signs that this may be happening. You may notice that your patience is short, that you're jittery, that your tone of voice is tinged with sarcasm, or that you're irritated by things that you usually would let pass. When you find this is so, take a break. Find someone to talk to. Get away. Otherwise, your anger can undo much of the good work you've done.

As we've pointed out, there's not much evidence that you're to blame for your child's eating disorder. However, there is growing evidence that you can be part of the solution, regardless of the cause of the eating disorder, but only if you aren't feeling guilty and powerless. Feeling guilty is especially problematic when you're trying to get started. Blaming yourself leads to a lot of second-guessing and hesitation on your part, which gives the eating disorder room to maneuver and slip through.

> Keshia felt sure that her own weight struggles and dieting were the cause of the bulimia nervosa that her 15-year-old daughter was struggling with. She felt that it was hypocritical to ask her daughter to eat regularly when she herself had for so many years dieted while her weight yo-yoed.

Keshia had a point—it probably wouldn't help for her to be dieting or worrying about her own weight when her daughter was struggling. But there was a difference. Keshia had never developed an eating disorder, whereas her daughter had. By blaming herself and holding back on doing what she could to help her daughter, Keshia was actually allowing bulimia to get a firmer grip on her child. Their family therapist pointed out that Keshia was hesitating and not following through on monitoring her daughter because of guilt. This was ultimately more harmful than anything she might have done before, because now her daughter needed her help. Keshia decided that even if she felt guilty, she would not let it interfere with helping her daughter. She found that helping her daughter actually lessened her guilt, especially as her daughter also began to respond.

FOCUS ON THE PROBLEM BEFORE YOU

As we suggested in Chapter 3, it's easy to become distracted and to be led down the primrose path if you spend a lot of time trying to figure out *why* your child developed an eating disorder. But there are many other ways to lose your way as well. Staying focused on what the problem is—disordered eating behaviors and beliefs—is challenging. To stay focused, it's imperative that you make changing disordered eating *the* priority, be available to intervene to change behaviors, establish a regular pattern of eating, and figure out ways to expand food choices, whether your child has anorexia, bulimia, or ARFID. At the same time, it's important to determine when it's reasonable to allow exercise, to prevent binge eating and purging, and to know when things are going well enough that you can begin to step back and hand control over eating back to your child. Let's examine each of these in turn to see how to stay focused.

Make Changing Disordered Eating Your Top Priority

To make changing disordered eating *the* priority sounds easy enough, but in practice families find this is harder than expected. In most families, plenty of distractions can and do interfere. The demands of work, household chores, needs of other family members, and so forth frequently command attention. For example, Laura's family was torn between her needs and those of her two siblings. Her parents felt it was unfair to pay such disproportionate attention to Laura and her problems. While this might be true, Laura was so malnourished that her life and future hung in the balance. Their therapist helped Laura's parents accept the fact that this extra focus on Laura was necessary but also see that it was *time limited*.

Danny's father was torn between his 13-year-old son's needs and his demanding job. As CEO of a large corporation, Danny's father traveled out of state almost weekly. Perhaps because Danny's mother was free to stay home and help their son fight anorexia nervosa, his father continued to make work his first priority. The family's therapist quickly stepped in and made a persuasive case for the need for the whole family to make changing Danny's disordered eating the number one priority. Danny's father was able to reschedule many of his upcoming trips and delegate his role to others in the company.

The demands of many professions can be compelling. And unlike Danny's family, many families will suffer financially when the parents take time off to help their child eat normally again. But for the sake of a child's continued survival and return to health, parents who take responsibility for their child's eating behaviors have to put that goal above all others. In addition, making this kind of intensive effort may appear costly at first, but in the long run it can prevent the need for even more expensive services, like hospital or residential treatment.

It's your therapist's task to help you keep this priority in focus and in your sights. You may be tempted to stray off into other "interesting issues," such as why the eating disorder arose in the first place, or to find "unavoidable obstacles" to taking charge, but these diversions will only keep you from the work you need to do at this point—getting your child to eat normally.

Be Available

By now you're undoubtedly getting the picture: You and/or your spouse will likely need to *be available* for all mealtimes and snacks to monitor eating at least for several weeks. This is a big adjustment for many parents, who have not been present for breakfast and lunch, or even dinner in some cases, sometimes for many years, because of work or school schedules. Accepting this requirement means that you will need to make adjustments to your personal and occupational lives. If the demands on your schedule seem onerous, go back to Chapter 1 and remind yourself that just because an eating disorder is a psychiatric illness does not mean that it is not serious. As we've shown, we see these illnesses as being on a par with any physical illness. They deserve to be given the same attention you would provide for a child after surgery, an accident, or another serious medical problem.

> Although it was a difficult decision, Jorge and Susan both took several weeks off from work to help Cindy. They discussed the pros and cons of this measure but ultimately decided that using sick leave and vacation time this way was necessary, as they now recognized how seriously ill Cindy was. Jorge had a harder time at first, and his boss was less sympathetic than Susan's. Jorge took some information about eating disorders and the treatment they were using to his boss. This helped her appreciate the gravity of Cindy's illness and Jorge's concern, as well as his need to be away from work more.

Don't assume you won't be able to negotiate a fair arrangement with your employer. Taking a brief medical leave is a good idea, because presenting a unified front at all meals is potentially most powerful, but in practical terms you may have to compromise. Figure out how you can adjust your schedule to allow you to be present at as many meals as possible. Maybe you can both plan to be on hand at breakfast and dinner but will have to alternate days off work to be present for lunch and snack times. A common solution in two-parent families is to divide up mealtimes, but this does leave each of you to battle the problem alone at different meals. As we discuss in Chapter 9, this can create a lot of opportunities for parents to drift into doing things differently at their respective mealtimes with the child, with the result that the eating disorder spots a chance to slip through the crack in the unified front. This is why we strongly encourage you to try to figure out from the start how both of you can be there at all meals, at least for the first few weeks.

If you have to split up the task, consider things such as whether one of you is more of a "morning person" than the other; in that case, the early riser could be assigned the job of making sure that breakfast is eaten. If only one of you can be available during the day, that one could go to school at snack and lunch times. Some parents have arranged for a school counselor or nurse to have lunch with their son or daughter, but this is usually appropriate only after some time has passed, once you have a plan that is generally working and you are getting sufficient cooperation from your child to try this. (There is more on figuring out when you can step back at the end of this chapter.)

If you don't have a spouse, it may be important to enlist the help of another adult relative. This can be effective even when two parents are available, as it was with Sarah, whose parents both worked but whose grandmother—who was the main cook in the house, in any event—was available at all mealtimes.

It may seem that your just being present won't make a big difference in terms of your child's eating, but it will. Being there provides both emotional and structural support, as well as encouragement to eat. Of course, your child won't benefit from this support and encouragement unless she too is present for all mealtimes. This sometimes means a leave from school or home study for several weeks, taken as a medical leave. This is often the preferred strategy, as it was in Cindy's case.

> Susan asked Cindy's pediatrician to write a note that would excuse Cindy from school for several weeks because of her medical and psychiatric fragility. Because this was clearly appropriate, the pediatrician provided the note and Cindy's schoolwork was brought to her by a home teacher on a weekly basis. Cindy fought this arrangement at first, claiming she would miss too much work. Her parents pointed out that at this point her health, not her schoolwork, was the priority. Although they also supported Cindy's academic achievements, they said good grades would be irrelevant if she did not recover from anorexia nervosa. This plan allowed Cindy and the family to focus on eating rather than on the social and academic pressures at school.

As noted earlier, sometimes parents are able to attend school during the lunch hour or work with the school to develop a flexible schedule for a few weeks to permit eating to take place at home. Understandably, most adolescents don't like their parents showing up at school to eat with them. It is, however, a reminder of the cost of the illness to them that they readily appreciate, so sometimes it's an additional motivation to the child to return to normal eating. Yet being at home for all meals can send a clear message about the importance of your child's health relative to academic work at this point in time, making it clear what the first priority is. You'll have to decide which will be a more powerful incentive for your child and help her make the needed changes.

Although this example focuses on the need to monitor eating in the case of anorexia nervosa, it's just as important that regular eating occur for children with bulimia, binge-eating disorder, or ARFID, as we have stressed; otherwise, they will retain the behaviors that are maintaining their eating disorder. So, your help in making sure that eating is monitored throughout the day, at least initially, is almost always necessary when using FBT for any eating disorder.

Besides both parents and the teenager with an eating disorder, siblings and other family members living at home need to be available for meals, too. Having the whole family eat together as much as possible definitely makes a difference, because that way your child knows that everyone is trying to help her. As parents, you help by making sure the right foods and the right amounts of food are prepared and eaten. Siblings help alleviate the tension and stress of trying to eat and contribute to making mealtimes more normal. They also distract the child with an eating disorder, to some extent, from thinking only about what she has to eat. They can also support her if she becomes angry or upset about your demands that she eat.

> Seventeen-year-old Todd had had a relatively close relationship with his sister, Cindy, when they were younger, but he was pretty busy with his own life now. He resented having to be home for dinner at first. His coach told him he might have to leave his basketball team if he missed too many practices, which often stretched into the dinner hour. Jorge and Susan worked hard to accommodate Todd's schedule because they thought he was important to helping Cindy. At first Cindy ignored Todd, but when she saw that he made such a big effort to be there, she turned to him more often for support when she felt overwhelmed by fighting with her parents.

Ballet lessons, soccer, and friends, among many other distractions, are likely to beckon and take your other children away from the table at mealtimes, so you will have to make a strong case for why everyone needs to be present and call on the assistance of the therapist to support your request. We stress that this need to be together for most meals will not last forever but that it's important now because a member of the family is ill and needs everyone's help. Usually, when brothers and sisters realize the urgency of getting their sibling to start eating normally or to stop purging, they acquiesce. But you should still be prepared to find ways to accommodate their needs, too. One family excused their other children from family dinners two nights during the week and in this way helped them be more supportive and less resentful of helping their sister with anorexia nervosa. It will be up to you to determine what's possible, keeping in mind the option of leaving a sibling out of the plan for a while if that child is so resentful about giving up the time or certain activities that his being at the table is completely counterproductive. Even in this case, though, you should continue to encourage all other siblings to participate. Many eventually do come around. For example, Darren, a 10-year-old boy whose sister Terry had anorexia, persisted in teasing and calling her names, but he started to change his tune after his parents recognized how jealous he was of the time they were spending with Terry and made an effort to address his needs as well.

This is a common problem, especially with younger siblings, who initially feel anxious and slighted because of the focus on a sibling with an eating disorder. It can be tough on parents to find a way to take care of all the needs of their children at once, but often, just spending a little focused time with the unaffected siblings helps reduce tension and jealousy.

Also be prepared for the fact that many siblings don't want to be involved because they simply feel they don't know how to help at first. Over time, if encouraged, they usually find ways to help that fit their relationships with their sibling.

At first, Todd was at a loss about what he could do to help. However, it soon became clearer that he didn't need to do anything dramatic. So, each week he would find something "nice" to do for Cindy. For example, he would ask her to play a video game (one of her choosing) after dinner or watch a video with her. As Cindy improved, he volunteered to go places with her and asked her to his games. This was enough for both Cindy and Todd. By being at the meals, Todd served as a comforting presence for his sister and a reminder that she had a relationship with someone, other than with her eating disorder.

Establish a Regular Pattern of Eating

Once you, your child with the eating disorder, and the rest of your family are able to be present during most meals, the next challenge is to structure those mealtimes throughout the day. Whether the disorder is anorexia nervosa, bulimia nervosa, binge-eating disorder, or ARFID, regular mealtimes are imperative. Again, this practice may diverge widely from what you were doing before the eating disorder developed. In our busy lives, meals are increasingly quick, eaten alone, and at haphazard times. In our experience of interviewing families, it is not uncommon at the beginning of treatment for families to have no set pattern for eating. What was pretty normal for many of these families when their children were quite young—three meals and two or three snacks—was no longer the case. So it may be a struggle at first to set up this mealtime structure again, but it is essential. In the case of anorexia nervosa, the body needs regular feeding to sustain itself physically. However, in addition, as many of those with the illness will tell you, if they skip eating for several hours, the desire to continue fasting increases. For those with bulimia nervosa and binge-eating disorder, skipping meals entails another hazard—increasing the risk of binge eating because of increased hunger—so in both cases structured eating times promote normalizing eating patterns. In Cindy's case, Susan and Jorge established regular mealtimes. Breakfast was at about 7:00 A.M., morning snack at about 10:00 A.M., lunch at noon, afternoon snack at 3:00 P.M., dinner at 6:00 P.M., and nighttime snack at 9:30 P.M. Similarly, children with ARFID often need a lot of structure and support at mealtimes to eat enough, try new foods, and overcome fears about eating. So regular mealtimes are helpful to establish new patterns that allow for consistent changes in eating behavior.

You may face some difficulties in trying to structure eating. The main obstacles are usually conflicting schedules for work, school, and other activities of siblings or parents. One mother, a nurse who worked the night shift, requested a change of schedule for several months. A father who had a long morning commute prepared breakfast for his wife and son and then left it for them. In this way he could contribute to the morning meal even though he wasn't there. To understand the importance of a regular meal schedule, it may be helpful to remember when your child was an infant and you had to feed her at regular and close intervals to ensure her health and growth. For most parents that was an exhausting and demanding time, but it lasted for only a year or so in most cases. That's what has to happen again here. The difference is that back then she probably cried to let you know she was hungry. Now her illness keeps her from crying out.

Related to the difficulty in setting up a schedule, a common impediment is travel. Travel during the early part of treatment is not usually a good idea. Travel means a change of schedules, eating in restaurants, and often stressful social situations for your child, who may not be ready for them, as was the case with Tamara.

> Tamara wanted to go to New York to visit relatives. She knew this would be hard, and she promised to eat, but when she got to New York she found that she couldn't. She didn't trust the restaurants, and she was not yet ready to eat with anyone other than her mother and father. When she returned, she had lost 6 pounds and was close to needing to be hospitalized because her heart rate had dropped perilously low.

Even a trip to Disneyland designed as a reward for progress can cause problems because such a reward, if it occurs too early, can backfire. The success that earned the trip can quickly disappear because of the limited availability of "safe foods" and "safe situations" for someone who is still early in recovery. Nonetheless, some travel may be necessary. When it is, parents have discovered that they need to be prepared by taking along a range of foods in case they find themselves in situations where the choices are not good or restaurants are too challenging. Sometimes this means an extra suitcase, but being prepared is well worth the inconvenience overall.

Once your child is starting to recover, brief trips can be a way of evaluating progress and promoting new experiments with eating that challenge the distorted assumptions about eating, food, and weight common to anorexia, bulimia, and ARFID. Often a good way to start is to visit "safe" or "comfortable" local restaurants to see how eating goes in these environments.

In rare instances, though, traveling can be helpful even early in treatment. One family that had enormous difficulty being together because of work and school found that when they spent 2 weeks in Hawaii, they could actually be available and support their daughter for the first time. They didn't eat out much. Still, when they returned to the mainland, they saw the progress that had been made, and this helped motivate them to keep at it even when they were home.

Help Your Child with Anorexia or ARFID Eat More

When recovering from anorexia nervosa or malnutrition related to ARFID, in contrast to bulimia nervosa or binge-eating disorder, your child has to eat not only regularly but also a lot. This is usually the next challenge after you've established a pattern of eating: how to increase the amount your child is eating.

> Using their schedule, Jorge and Susan tried to determine what they thought Cindy should eat at each meal and snack. At first they asked the therapist to tell them what she should eat. The therapist said she was confident they would figure out how to feed Cindy. She pointed out that Cindy's older brother, Todd, was a healthy high school senior. The therapist explained that the reason she could not tell them what to do was that Jorge and Susan were the ones who had to carry out whatever plan they came up with. The therapist said she would be happy to advise them, based on her experience. She said sometimes parents didn't at first appreciate how much more their child with anorexia needed to eat. It was important to remember that

gaining weight requires more eating than just maintaining weight.

Like Cindy's parents, you may find it a challenge to decide how much food to provide to your malnourished child at each meal. Parents typically find themselves underestimating how much their child needs to eat. We've often heard parents say, "How can she not be gaining weight? She's eating more than I do!" But what parents sometimes fail to see is that a person who is malnourished is actually burning food extremely rapidly, and not until rather large quantities are consumed is it possible to make headway.

Getting your child to eat more when she thinks she doesn't want to is at the heart of the challenge of recovering from these disorders. There are lots of ways parents succeed, but first they must set *clear expectations*. Veronica's parents set out her complete meals and snacks, based on the amounts they thought she needed to eat to recover her weight loss. They would put the food she was to eat on her plate. She had absolutely no choice in what she ate or the amount. Her parents knew from experience that offering Veronica a choice put her in a predicament she couldn't yet resolve: to give up anorexia nervosa or keep it. Veronica did not like this, of course, but another part of her was somewhat relieved that she didn't have to decide. If they make me eat, she thought, I can't be held responsible. This would temporarily relieve the anxiety and stress she felt about eating and gaining weight. Sarah's parents did it a little differently. They felt that Sarah could fill her plate and choose what to eat, but they also made it clear that if they thought what she chose was insufficient, they would add to it.

For some parents, offering limited choices works well, as long as they are the ones who decide whether the amount is sufficient. Of course, if just setting the right expectations and filling plates were enough, we probably would not need to write this book. In addition to providing enough food, you have to establish *clear consequences* for not eating.

Veronica knew that if she did not eat, she would have to stay in her room on her bed, where she could read or do homework, but no other distractions would be permitted. She also knew that if she persisted in not eating, her parents would take her to the pediatrician, who would ultimately admit her to the hospital if her heart rate or her body temperature was too low, where she would have to stay until she was better. She knew that if that happened she would be made to eat there.

As we mentioned earlier when we talked about blame, setting consequences can help you avoid the trap of responding angrily to food refusal. This is why consequences should be established well ahead of time, certainly before the plate is on the table. Again, each family must decide on the best way to impose consequences.

Sarah's parents decided not to impose consequences for failure to eat a certain amount at an individual meal. Instead, they would praise Sarah for what she did eat, ignore what she did not, but make it clear that they hoped she would do better. It was at the end of the day that they would make it clear to Sarah that if she didn't continue to gain weight, they would need to become stricter. This meant that they would offer fewer choices and allow less freedom.

An important factor to keep in mind about consequences is that for most families these are really protections for the child. Viewing them this way may make it easier for you to impose them and for your child to accept them. When your child is malnourished, it may sound and feel like punishment to your daughter to have to stay in bed and rest, but when she is malnourished it is also *necessary*, to make sure she doesn't lose more weight through exertion. Similarly, keeping your son out of school may seem unfair and counterproductive, but school, though a source of accomplishment for many, is often actually stressful and adds to the burden of trying to fight the disordered thinking associated with an eating disorder.

Reasonable, productive consequences may also help you avoid harsher punishments, which are rarely helpful. Parents sometimes entertain the idea of imposing harsh punishments for not eating because eating disorders can be such frustrating illnesses. Most parents avoid resorting to such measures because they already, correctly, see their child as sensitive and generally responsive to gentler correctives—at least in everything except eating. In most cases, even those who try harsher punishments quickly find them counterproductive, leading to a hardening of their child's resolve against their efforts to gain the child's cooperation.

After being clear about both what you expect and what will happen if your expectations aren't met, the next challenge is *sticking with it* and being doggedly persistent. This is where you must outlast the willful hold the eating disorder has on your child. Remember, you have several advantages. First, in situations where there are two parents, at least when you are working together, your combined energy can thwart the eating disorder more effectively. In this instance, two against one (when the one is anorexia or bulimia) is fair play. Next, you are older and wiser and more experienced. You know your child and what makes her tick. You can use that information to slowly build motivation to fight anorexia within her. Moreover, even if your child is an adolescent, you continue to have both legal and parental authority to count on. These are no small advantages, inasmuch as they can allow you to make decisions on behalf of your child even when the teenager, because of her illness, refuses to cooperate with interventions like going to therapy or being admitted to a hospital. You also love your child, and your dedication to her welfare supplies a powerful reservoir of energy for you to call on when you're struggling.

Regardless of these advantages, you still will need to outlast, outmaneuver, and overcome the eating disorder. Like any plan, it is only a plan until and if it is *carried out*. This is where parents usually have the most difficulty. They want it to be easier, they want it be shorter, and sometimes they want someone else to do it. Carrying out the plan and consequences is the *work* that must be done, and there's no getting around it. Your patience, energy, and determination will all be tried. We like to remind parents that eating disorders don't develop overnight; instead, they begin, as we described in Chapter 1, insidiously and slyly. We like to remind parents that eating disorders must be defeated *one bite at a time.*

It might help if you think of carrying out the plan like weeding an overgrown garden. If at the beginning of the day you focus on how many weeds there are and how long it will take and how tiring the job is, you will have trouble getting past the first few feet. Instead, just starting to weed, pulling out weeds one by one, and focusing on that single weed that's rooted deeply, then moving on to the next, slowly but perceptibly, you will make progress. So, Julia's parents felt dismayed and defeated when they had only gotten Julia to eat two or three more bites of bland fish than she had the day before. They wanted to give up. They felt incompetent and angry. The therapist working with them encouraged them to see it another way. He said, "You have succeeded in helping Julia eat three bites she otherwise would not have. That is a great start. If she eats six bites tomorrow, that's better still. Hang in there." Treading the line between being clear about expectations and being flexible enough to find alternatives, while also not giving in to the eating disorder, is tricky business. While not completely overwhelming your child, you have to make it impossible for the eating disorder to slip through.

> Over the next several days, every meal Cindy ate was an ordeal. Susan and Jorge talked together after each attempt and tried to identify new ways to encourage their daughter. First they tried to bribe her: "If you eat this, we'll get you that new laptop." Cindy did eat, but she stopped again at the next meal. "It wasn't worth it," she said. Next they tried making her feel guilty: "Look how upset everyone is. Your mother can't sleep nights. We are all a wreck!" This made Cindy cry, and she tried to eat but ended up just feeling worse. What did appear to work was saying very little about eating or food. Just encouraging her to keep trying and making sure she rested and had little other stress or distractions seemed to be helpful. Little by little their patience and persistence began to show results. Cindy's resolve not to eat slowly began to crumble in the face of their loving determination. First it was a mouthful of chicken, then a half cup of milk, but the progress was steady, and when the family met with the therapist and saw that Cindy was gaining weight, albeit slowly at first, they had their first taste of hope for many months.

You will often be told by your child that she's "too full" or her "stomach hurts" or she's "not hungry" and that she's "just eaten." In a way, each of these statements may contain a grain of truth, but they miss the point. For anorexia nervosa, eating more than usual is necessary. In the case of anorexia and sometimes ARFID, food is literally medicine. Parents can, however, help their child with these complaints to a limited extent. One set of parents found that it helped their son to drink a liquid supplement rich in nutrition (proteins and essential fatty acids) as a regular part of his meals because it made him feel less full as well as reduced his discomfort after eating. It was also a rich source of calories. Other parents have found it helpful to make sure enough is eaten early in the day so they can be a little more flexible later on. Sometimes, something as simple as a heating pad or hot water bottle, a gentle neck rub, or another soothing activity helps, because it is really not the physical problem that is causing discomfort (though it seems to your child that it is), but more the emotional discomfort she feels about eating and the anxiety she has about gaining weight that's at the root of her complaints.

We often use the metaphor of "climbing a sand hill" to describe how one must proceed in this refeeding effort. When climbing a sand hill, you have to keep moving up the hill, or the loose sand will cause you to slip back down. If you keep moving up the hill at a sufficiently quick pace, you will find you can proceed, with effort, toward your destination. However, if you pause to rest, you begin to slide and may find yourself back where you started. Only when you've reached the top of the hill can you rest.

Help Your Child with Anorexia or ARFID Expand Food Choices

In addition to structuring eating times and helping your child eat more, it's important to help your child expand the types of foods she will eat. Children with eating disorders have often developed a very specific list of foods they feel comfortable eating. Often these foods are very low-calorie, non- or low-fat, and low-density foods. Or, as is the case with bulimia nervosa and binge-eating disorder, there are foods that they crave (often candies, starches, breads), but they allow themselves only small amounts—until a binge episode occurs. In either case, the children's preoccupations with food choices are also further delimited by calorie counting, fat gram counting, weighing and measuring food, demands that they prepare all food for themselves (and sometimes others), and sometimes the use of specific cooking pots, plates, bowls, or utensils.

You will have to decide whether you want to approach this range of behaviors as one big problem area—in which case you might just decide what and how your child should eat, as you did when he was much younger. This means that you wouldn't permit calorie counting (or at least not base what was being eaten on a specific caloric amount); you would insist on fat consumption and require that a range of food be eaten. You see, unless challenged, each of these behaviors encourages the persistence of eating-disordered thinking. Counting calories means setting a constant measure (one that the "dieting" teenager will always wish to be lower) by which to evaluate eating. The same goes for fat grams, as well as measuring and weighing portions. In other words, this obsessiveness about food measurement reinforces disordered thinking about food. This is true of all food rules in general. The rules that the person with an eating disorder sets up appear at first to protect him from overeating and gaining weight, but such rules ultimately backfire and become a cage of regulations that prevent normal eating. So, when you challenge these rules, you are challenging the disordered thinking about food that underlies the disorders.

It can be argued that a full-scale assault on this disordered thinking is the best way to proceed, and it is the basis of many hospital and residential refeeding programs. Yet you might feel, as many parents do, that you want to take a more gradual approach to changing these behaviors. Thus, you may want to start by allowing some of the food rules to persist if eating improves and weight gain is appropriate in the case of anorexia or ARFID. If you take this approach, you may experience a bit less resistance about eating from your child at first, but you will be in for a longer haul.

> Gia's parents decided they would ask her to eat one new food a week. The *amount* she ate would be what she needed to continue to make progress on her weight gain, but in addition, she could choose one new food to add to her diet—usually a food that was one she was struggling with but in the past enjoyed. In Gia's case the first food to be added was cheese. She had always

liked cheese but had become completely unwilling to eat it over the past 6 months because she was afraid of the fat it contained. Gia's parents gave her a choice about *what* cheese she was going to start with, *but she had to choose one.* Gia chose Parmesan cheese. She felt more comfortable with that because it was shredded and seemed less threatening (or fattening) as a result. She sprinkled only a little on her salad, but she tried it. Again, the process was slow at first, but gradually she became used to eating Parmesan cheese and was more willing to try other cheeses as well.

Another challenge that arises fairly frequently is drinking whole milk. Most adolescents who are malnourished refuse to drink whole milk. "Too much fat," they say. But fat is what many of them need, so getting them to switch from nonfat milk to whole milk (even if just for a time) can provide an important source of nutrition. "Pick your battles" is our usual advice to parents about food choices. Don't argue over a lettuce leaf. Argue over something that counts—fettuccine with cream sauce or steak and mashed potatoes. Whole milk may or may not be worth fighting for if your child's diet already contains enough calcium and fat. Whitney's parents thought it was worth the battle, and they simply didn't buy nonfat or low-fat milk. This was a switch for the family (and one that was only temporary, until Whitney was better nourished). At first Whitney balked, but when her parents gently but relentlessly prodded her, she gave in. In the beginning she took only a little milk on cereal, then a half cup with a snack, but in the end the part of Whitney that knew she needed to drink milk to get better began to submit, and she actually slowly agreed that it was a good idea—at least until she was at a healthy weight.

Help Your Child Use Exercise Appropriately

Exercise is a wonderful thing. However, in the minds of those with eating disorders, it can become an opportunity to express a great deal of pathology. In those with anorexia nervosa, exercise is an effective way to lose weight and to keep from gaining weight. In those with bulimia nervosa, exercise is sometimes used as a way of purging by making sure that any calories consumed are balanced by calories exercised away on a treadmill or bike.

It's often challenging to know how and when to intervene in relation to exercise. Certainly, if your child has anorexia nervosa and is underweight, exercise should generally be prohibited. This means letters to school (sometimes requiring a physician's note as well) exempting your child from physical education. Sometimes it means monitoring in-room exercising (sit-ups, jumping jacks, and so forth). Again, your involvement is aimed at promoting the physical health of your child rather than allowing continued deterioration. So, as soon as your child is eating normally and out of medical danger, it's usually a good idea to allow exercising, in moderation, once again. As with eating, however, you may at first have to be scrupulous about this reintroduction, as it's very easy for your child to get carried away. Hence, it's helpful to lay out a careful plan. For example, you could allow 15 minutes of exercise a day to begin with, and if weight continues to improve, this can be increased to 30 minutes, where it should probably remain until all signs of the disorder are gone. In some cases it's helpful to allow exercise a bit earlier. Some parents have found this helps improve appetite, support cooperation, and increase motivation for recovery. We think that this approach can indeed be helpful, but only if you and the medical professionals you are working with feel comfortable with it. Practically, this usually means that your child is continuing to show progress in regard to her eating and weight.

For those with bulimia nervosa and binge-eating disorder, reasonable exercise, not in relation to overeating or binge eating, can help minimize frustration and increase tolerance for not purging. Often, the child may resort to purging in lieu of exercise because exercising is perceived as being more work and taking more time. Helping your child with bulimia nervosa develop a reasonable, structured approach to exercise, very similar to that taken in structuring meals, can offset this perception. Sometimes joining a health club or a structured exercise program (kickboxing, karate, and so forth) in which thinness is not a virtue works well. (Some types of dance classes, in which a slim appearance seems to matter, can backfire.) You may want to help your child identify a friend to exercise with so she'll be more likely to stick with it. Depending on the nature of your relationship with your child, you may even be able to act as your child's exercise partner. Either way, your encouragement about this way of attaining and maintaining a healthy weight and body can be very beneficial for those with bulimia.

Help Your Child Prevent Binge Eating and Purging

In addition to everything we've already said about normalizing eating, you'll need to prevent binge eating and purging when your child's problem includes these behaviors. In the case of binge eating, for example, you are primarily responsible for what foods are available and when they are available to be consumed in your home. Therefore, it helps a great deal for you to understand more about *what* foods are likely to lead to your child's binge eating. These foods vary from person to person, but it is usually pretty evident from what's missing from your cabinets which foods your child is likely to binge eat. Common examples are cereal (by the box), ice cream (by the half gallon), and whole packages of cookies, potato chips, and cheese, and jars of peanut butter. A general rule is that binge foods are typically high-calorie, high-fat, and often sweet foods—foods that dieters try hard to limit severely and that therefore represent an indulgence.

One teenager reported that her mother routinely baked a cake for dessert on Sunday. Each member of the family of four had a piece, leaving half a cake. This cake was a consistently available and desirable food to binge on each Sunday evening. Another child reported that the "stock" of large bags of potato chips and ice cream containers bought at wholesale food markets and stored in the pantry and refrigerator were a constant source of binge foods. It's perfectly understandable that you'll sometimes bake cakes or that you might be in the habit of buying food in bulk to economize. Until your child is in better control of binge eating, however, you may need to change these and similar ways of cooking and shopping. There are likely other ways in which you're supplying foods that lend themselves to binge eating that you might curtail for the time being.

In addition to making tempting foods available, you may be unwittingly supporting binge eating by not being present to prevent it. Many binge eaters will do so only in private because they're ashamed of the behavior. So, many teenagers who binge eat figure

Taking Charge of Change

out the times when no one is likely to be around or when their activities will go undetected. There are usually several such times each day. One is after school between 3:00 and 6:00 P.M., and other times are late at night or very early in the morning. These times also fit nicely into the distorted eating pattern that usually accompanies bulimia nervosa, because long periods of "restricting"—all day or all night, for example—produce increased hunger and feelings of deprivation, leading, in response, to overeating during a binge. So it is very important that you become aware of the most likely periods when your child will binge eat and that you make an effort to be available during those times to help prevent the behavior.

With bulimia nervosa, most purging follows the consumption of a lot of food, precipitated by guilt, shame, and anxiety about overeating and fear of gaining weight. Purging, like binge eating, is usually a secretive behavior. Because purging is effective only in emptying undigested food (to the limited degree that it is) only fairly soon (usually within 30 minutes) after eating, it is a considerably predictable behavior. So, if you know *when* your child has eaten, or particularly when he has binge eaten, you are in a position to know when he will try to purge. Thus, as in the case of binge eating, knowing the time purging is likely to occur will help you know when to be on the lookout and to implement strategies to prevent it.

It's also helpful to know *where* your child purges. This is not always so straightforward. Most, of course, purge into the toilet, but many also purge in the shower, into garbage bags, or into shrubbery. Purging is often governed by very specific rules—and can be done only under those conditions. For example, some people can purge only at home, others can purge only when no one is around, and others have rules about where they cannot purge, such as at school or at church. When these conditions are understood, it is much easier to prevent them from being met and thereby disallow the opportunity for purging. If your child purges only at home (which is not uncommon in the early stages of the illness), you have an advantage because you have a specific limited environment to monitor. Nonetheless, the conditions can change, and it's important to keep abreast of any changes in locations for purging because any change opens a potential loophole to allow the behavior to continue.

It is also important to learn about *how* your child purges. Most often this simply involves putting a finger down the throat, stimulating a gag reflex. However, sometimes this is ineffective and other instruments, such as spoons, toothbrushes, nail files, and so forth, are used. Some adolescents learn about syrup of ipecac, which is used to cause emesis after poisoning. When used routinely to purge, however, it is associated with cardiac problems and even death. Over time, some people learn to purge without any direct stimulation. This means that it's possible to purge at any time and very surreptitiously, making the behavior more difficult to detect and disrupt. Nonetheless, knowledge of the means your child uses to purge will help you intervene, because you can look for the signs of continued purging activity (for example, broken nails, scratches on the back of the hand from teeth scratching it). If your child uses syrup of ipecac, it's essential that you remove this substance from your home or lock it up because of the danger it poses.

Remember, your child will feel compelled to purge if she believes she's overeaten (and in this sense, she has little choice about her wish). Furthermore, she feels tremendous relief if she purges. Thus, purging is a very reinforcing behavior, even if it is shameful and sometimes painful. Your job is to help her tolerate the discomfort of not purging while supplying other positive reinforcements instead of purging, such as attention, distractions, or opportunities for other positive things to do. *To provide these alternatives, you need to talk to your child about what she thinks would be helpful.* Some parents have found playing a video game, watching a movie, taking a walk, or going shopping may help prevent purging when a period of binge eating has occurred.

Laxative abuse is another common way that some adolescents attempt to purge their foods. As we noted in Chapter 4, taking laxatives is a very dangerous way to go about this and is very ineffective, in addition. The use of laxatives over the long term leads to a variety of medical problems, including severe abdominal pain, bloating, and intestinal plasticity. To be effective, doses have to be increased, which can result in toxicity in some cases. Many who use laxatives report that they wish to feel "empty" and to "flatten their stomachs" rather than just get rid of food. Psychologically, emptying the gut feels like a relief as well. To help your child stop taking laxatives, keep several things in mind. Certain laxatives can be detected in blood or stool samples, and your pediatrician can test for those, helping you know whether your child is using them without your knowledge. In addition, laxatives can be expensive if used frequently, so if your child has a ready supply of cash, you should monitor spending to make sure it isn't being used to purchase laxatives. However, many adolescents also steal laxatives because of their cost. It is not uncommon for persons with bulimia to be caught shoplifting laxatives.

Purging can also take the form of extreme exercise. After binge eating, your child may try to estimate the number of calories she consumed and try to "run it off" on a treadmill or through other strenuous activities. This pattern of exercise purging may not appear to be as harmful as taking laxatives or vomiting, but because of the stress it places on the body, as well as the anxiety about "not getting all the calories worked off" and the time it takes, trying to compensate for a binge through exercise can exact a great toll. Your role in such a situation is to help your child exercise as a usual activity for health, not weight control per se, and especially not to compensate for abnormal binge eating, which results from unduly restrictive dieting.

DON'T DEBATE WITH YOUR CHILD ABOUT EATING- OR WEIGHT-RELATED CONCERNS

One of the most common problems parents face, and you probably will too, is the distorted thinking of the child with an eating disorder. You may believe that you should be able to get your child to "see reason," "be reasonable," or "see the light" or that she "will just get over it." At the start, this just doesn't happen very often (if at all). Instead, what happens is that you are often drawn into a variety of debates and struggles that are illogical from start to finish, except from the perspective of someone whose thinking is distorted with overconcern about, unrealistic investment in, and anxiety about food, weight, and shape. We discussed in detail what this thinking is like in Chapter 5. However, when you're in the trenches, up against anorexia, bulimia, or ARFID, the problems that this thinking can cause you are no longer abstract; they are quite specific, and it's not always clear how to proceed. Examples of the difficulties you will face include obsessive weighing, food shopping, clothes shopping, the influence of friends, and the influence of the media and fashion.

Don't Permit Obsessive Weighing

Constant weighing is a common problem in many people with eating disorders. There is an obsessional quality to it, so much so that over time weighing becomes a way of assessing their emotional state (feeling good or bad), their self-worth (successful or a failure), and their desirability (being likable or unlikable). Of course, a person's weight does not really define these attributes, but their association with weighing over time makes it seem so. In addition, weighing at really frequent intervals is deceptive and inaccurate. Too many other factors (what the person is wearing, when the person ate, time of day, recent activity, recent fluid intake) can change weight by 1–3 pounds. You will notice that your child may be momentarily reassured by a low weight, only to come crashing down a few hours later because of a "high" weight. You know her weight has not changed substantially, but that's not how it feels to your child. At the same time, it's important that weight be taken at regular intervals so that everyone knows how things are progressing. For all these reasons, we recommend that during treatment weight be taken only once or twice a week. This may mean throwing out the bathroom scale (or hiding it). It is also useful if the professionals you work with agree on when weight will be taken and who will take it. There's nothing helpful about a child's weight going up in the pediatrician's office, down in the nutritionist's office, and being unchanged in the therapist's office. Having too many scales just leaves everyone confused.

Decide When It Is a Good Idea to Take Your Child Grocery Shopping

Shopping for food when your child has an eating disorder can be a very difficult proposition. There will be a lot of rules you're supposed to follow, and these rules tend to change a lot. Still, some parents elect to take their child with them when shopping to help them buy foods that the child will agree to eat. In our experience, this is often counterproductive. The child wanders the grocery store aisles looking for something acceptable to eat (but finding very little) if she has anorexia nervosa, and feeling guilty and tempted if she has bulimia nervosa or binge-eating disorder. So, early in treatment, though it is good to understand your child's likes and dislikes, it is often better to shop alone. Later, once recovery has started, involving your child in these excursions is useful as it allows you and the child to better see the progress being made in terms of comfort with food and more flexibility in her choices.

Hold Off Clothes Shopping Until Symptoms Are Decreased

Shopping for clothes, another common activity for teenagers, is best limited during the early part of treatment as well. Often, like weight, clothing sizes will serve as "markers" for emotional and social worth. A child's pride in being size 0 is as distorted as the shame in being size 20 in the context of an eating disorder. Overall, though, because the size that fits an adolescent with anorexia nervosa will be increasing, it just makes sense to wait until full (or nearly full) weight recovery before shopping for clothes. For those with bulimia nervosa, the issue is often one of sizes going up and down during the period of early treatment, meaning that here too it's better to wait.

One shopping trip you may not be able to avoid is the one for a special outfit, such as for a dance, particularly a dress for a girl. Such dresses and occasions often stimulate much anxiety on everyone's part. Be sure to evaluate your own investment in this process inasmuch as fashion and appearance affect us all. Try to avoid dresses that are too form fitting, regardless of how stylish, because they tend to emphasize many of the characteristics, for good or ill, that your child worries so much about.

Allow Supportive Friendships

Parents often worry about whether a friend who has an eating disorder will have a negative impact on their child's progress. There is no simple answer to this question because so much depends on the friend and your child. A great number of teenagers have eating disorders, so it is likely you won't be able to avoid them. If, however, your child's friend is not being treated and also appears to be encouraging eating-disordered behaviors in your child, it would be wise to limit this friendship as much as possible, at least during the early period of treatment. This is a delicate problem, though, because teenagers' friends are very important to them. If you feel it is absolutely necessary to limit contact with a particular friend, be clear about your reasons and about your intention to reevaluate the situation as your child continues to make progress. Certainly, it is important to discuss this significant issue with your child's therapist to get further guidance.

Limit the Influence of Media-Related Values Regarding Weight

A number of influences beyond your home and family will affect how your child thinks about herself. Some of these influences are general and touch all of us in one way or another (for example, media, fashion, and culture); others are peculiar to the adolescent world (adolescent peer groups and values), and some to the world of eating disorders (pro–eating disorder websites). How can you limit the negative aspects of these external influences insofar as they may keep your child from fully recovering from an eating disorder?

Adolescents are particularly vulnerable to the influences of media. They are still developing a sense of who they are and are seeking outside confirmation for their emerging identities. Ironically, in a sense, adolescents often seek to conform to a set of norms as defined by the media rather than finding their own niches. This decision to conform has to do with the need to "fit in" with a peer group. Fitting in with a peer group is important for several reasons. First, as social animals, humans naturally seek out others. During adolescence, relationships outside the family constitute the vehicle whereby social learning, including dating, takes place. As a result, adolescents invest heavily in their peer groups. They want to be liked, and this may take on a very simple and concrete meaning for them: Being thin (or thinner) will make them more likable. It's easy to understand why adolescents see things this way—there's a certain degree of truth to this perception. However, they often fail to see that this is hardly the sole basis for being valued. Someone is more often liked because of being funny, smart, or kind. In addition, adolescents are still developing a sense of perspective. They turn to the media and their various products to help them see things outside their smaller world. Unfortunately, the popular media, on the whole, do not provide a real perspective, but instead a highly distorted one, where beauty and attractiveness define success, happiness, and accomplishment.

As a parent, it's your responsibility to help reestablish other values. When we talk to adolescents with eating disorders, we sometimes ask them to rank the relative importance of their weight or shape as compared with other attributes or concerns. Those with eating disorders substantially overvalue their weight and shape as compared with their intelligence, personality, friends, family, and even religious beliefs. Of course, weight is important for both health and attractiveness, but when it is *so* important that it substantially outranks all these other important qualities and relationships, it becomes a problem. It's more difficult for your child to see these other values, particularly in the visual media. The media cannot place values on these other factors—for one thing, they're harder to capture in a picture—and even if they did, these things wouldn't "sell" because they are unfortunately not perceived as "rare" or "special" the way beauty is.

As a parent of an adolescent, you are in a difficult position. You are an adult, and as such you are "out of touch," as it were (or as it seems), with the world of your teenager. If you directly question particulars in fashion (leggings, ripped jeans, spandex tops, and so forth), you will likely be dismissed. Therefore, it's important to approach the matter with more of a questioning attitude than a critical one. This means that if you want to help your child consider heroes or heroines outside the celebrity group, it's important to try to understand what other values your child holds that you might be able to tap into to encourage her in those directions. For example, if your child values academic or athletic achievement, these can be supported as alternatives to physical beauty in terms of value. It's also often possible to tap into the altruistic sentiments of many adolescents by identifying ways in which social values are opportunities for balancing the relative merits of physical attractiveness with other sources of self-esteem and self-worth, such as volunteering, tutoring, conservation programs, and religious and church groups.

The need for parents to respond to a child's overvaluing of appearance and attractiveness is not unique to parents whose children have eating disorders. However, you have a special task because your child has developed specific problems that play into the worst aspects of the physical ideals set up to be admired. Your mandate is to monitor and limit the influence of the values being promoted, at the same time identifying alternative sources and supporting your child in turning to them for the development of self-esteem and values.

Sometimes the media communicating health issues are even more problematic than the media promoting fashion and celebrity. This is the case, in part, because it is difficult to see health as a problematic value. What is problematic is the way health is defined. For example, there is frequent emphasis on vegetarianism, low-fat/nonfat foods, dieting, and certain kinds of intensive exercise regimens. In the hands (and head) of someone with an eating disorder, the worth of these things is exaggerated way out of reasonable proportion. We stress that most of these choices, when made in pursuit of health, lead to good outcomes, but when they are desired in order to diet or maintain an extremely low body weight, they do not.

Among the most insidious forces that now encroach on the health of adolescents with eating disorders are pro–eating disorder websites. These websites, cleverly labeled to be misleading, provide chat groups, information, and strategies that encourage adolescents to develop eating disorders, refuse intervention, and oppose parental involvement in their treatment. There is no easy solution. Free speech is guaranteed. However, as a parent you do have some options. It may seem draconian, but for the period of time that your child is in treatment, it may be necessary to disconnect his tablet, laptop, and smart phone from the internet or to allow it to be used only under very close supervision. You can learn techniques for detecting your adolescent's use of such sites—tracking "cookies"—but as is often the case, your child may be more savvy about digital media than you. Still, the perniciousness of these sites is so strong that we recommend taking a firm stance against accessing them by whatever means you have at your disposal. Of course, your adolescent may be able to access these sites from other venues (school, library, or friends), but the time he has will be more limited.

KNOW WHEN TO BEGIN BACKING OFF

As hard as it may be to imagine now, there will come a time when you will need to figure out how to begin backing off from being so involved in the day-to-day management of your child's eating disorder symptoms and behaviors. In fact, that is the ultimate goal of your getting so involved in the first place. You will know you're approaching that point when your child is at or very near her normal weight, is eating reasonable amounts on a reasonable schedule, is not compulsive in exercising, is not binge eating or purging, and is generally more like her old self. If your daughter lost her menstrual period, its return is also a very good indicator of physical health.

It can be difficult to let go after you have struggled so hard to get a hold on this problem. It's a frightening experience to see someone whose life you treasure veer off in a dangerous direction. Studies of childhood cancer survivors have shown that the kids who went through all the chemotherapy, radiation, and surgeries were, at a later point, not particularly preoccupied with those events. Yet their parents still had many worries, intrusive thoughts, dreams, and continued anxieties about what their child went through long before. So keep in mind that your child may move on and feel out of danger (and may even be right about this) before you feel comfortable again.

With regard to your starting to hand control back to your child, we often use the analogy of how you might manage letting your child drive again after a traffic infraction. You might start by allowing him to drive only to and from school, then later allowing him to drive in the daytime on weekends, and so on, until full privileges have been earned. With respect to eating, you might start with allowing your teenager to eat snacks unmonitored, then lunches, and so on, until you are confident that eating is going well without your supervision.

This may take several months to accomplish fully. Usually, by this time, you are more comfortable and know what to look for and how to help if problems arise.

We strongly encourage you, though, to try to allow as many other social activities as possible as your child is beginning to recover. We suggest that you do this—in part, because such engagements permit more normal development—while also ensuring that eating takes place. This may mean having to schedule activities after or before mealtimes when you're first getting started. Still, by encouraging these activities, you will be able to help your child see you as controlling only her eating behaviors and not interfering as much with other age-appropriate activities. Such an approach may also help your child tolerate your involvement in the area of eating.

We like to say that the ultimate goal in treating an eating disorder is to have *life* replace the obsessional behaviors and the thoughts about food and weight associated with them. For your adolescent, this means returning to school, taking up the challenge of explaining to her friends where she's been, and slowly entering a more normal adolescent social life. Returning to school is a worry, as the need to perform at high levels is so common to many with eating disorders. Because they've been ill, they feel they are behind and less well prepared, and perhaps they will never achieve what they hope to. Helping a child get back to school requires, in part, accepting the idea that some of this concern is okay. The thought to convey is "you can still be a good student, catch up, and be successful even if you don't take five AP [advanced placement] classes in your junior year." It requires a bit more tact or judgment to decide how much information about why the child has been out of school is appropriate to share. Most teenagers just say they had "heart problems" or "stomach problems" or something to that effect. Others, like Cindy, decide they want to help others through their experience. They become peer health aides who try to help other people with eating problems.

You may find that you need to help get your adolescent back on track by encouraging him more actively than you might have expected to. You may sometimes even have to take the lead in arranging visits with friends and encouraging attendance at school functions. Many children with eating disorders have some degree of social anxiety.

This may have to be addressed even after the eating-disordered behavior and thinking have subsided. Treatment for these problems, as for other psychiatric difficulties, such as depression or obsessive–compulsive disorder, may require separate treatment with medications, therapy, or both.

TAKE CARE OF YOURSELF

It was probably evident to you as you read this chapter that helping your child will be a lot of work. So it's important that while you're doing this crucial job you take care of yourself as much as possible. If you're not able to continue to support your child, she will lose her most important asset in her fight against her eating disorder. To take care of yourself, you must recognize that you will need more rest, regular exercise, and good nutrition. You should also plan on sharing the burden with your spouse and with other family members when you need a break. If you find yourself feeling depressed or overanxious, consider seeking additional personal therapy for support. In our experience, it has not been at all unusual for parents to seek such support. You may also find support through your family, friends, or spiritual community. Making use of your own support system will help both you and your child.

At the end of all this work, though, will be the great satisfaction that you have helped your child with a life-threatening problem. Although we cannot guarantee the outcome, as we have stated before, there's very good reason to be optimistic about your chances.

FOR MORE INFORMATION

Le Grange, D., and J. Lock, Bulimia Nervosa in Adolescents: Treatment, Eating Pathology, and Comorbidity, *South African Psychiatry Review,* 2002, 5, 19–22.

Le Grange, D., and J. Lock, *Treating Bulimia in Adolescents: A Family-Based Approach,* 2007. New York: Guilford Press.

Le Grange, D., J. Lock, and M. Dymek, Family-Based Therapy for

Adolescents with Bulimia Nervosa, *American Journal of Psychotherapy,* 2003, *67,* 237–251.

Le Grange, D., K. L. Loeb, S. Van Orman, et al., Bulimia Nervosa in Adolescents: A Disorder in Evolution?, *Archives of Pediatrics and Adolescent Medicine,* 2004, *158,* 478–482.

Lock, J., *Family-Based Treatment for Avoidant/Restrictive Food Intake Disorder,* 2022. New York: Routledge.

Lock, J., and D. Le Grange, *Treatment Manual for Anorexia Nervosa: A Family-Based Approach, Third Edition,* 2025. New York: Guilford Press.

Lock, J., A. Whyte, B. Matheson, and N. Datta, *Family-Based Treatment for Eating Disorders Piece by Piece: A Practical Guide for Parents,* 2024. New York: Routledge.

CHAPTER 8

Playing a Supporting Role

Other Ways You Can Be a Part of Your Child's Recovery

In Chapter 7 we focused on ways you can be involved in *directly* changing disordered eating and related behaviors through family-based treatment (FBT). In this chapter we illustrate how you can be involved in other types of treatment as well. The treatments discussed in this chapter were not developed with the tenets used in FBT in mind, and they vary in their adaptability to parental involvement. How much you are permitted and encouraged to participate may also vary from practitioner to practitioner within the same form of therapy. But all these therapies can be delivered in ways that do not exclude you, that show respect and support for your role as parents, that educate you about what is being done to help your child, and that specify how you *can* help. Your involvement in these other therapies is just as important as in family treatment, though your role in changing behaviors is usually more *indirect*.

In earlier chapters we emphasized that the importance of parents in supporting child and adolescent development has been underestimated. Increasingly, it is clear that involved parents make a real difference in how successfully children and teenagers negotiate their lives. So, whether you take a direct or an indirect role in helping your child, your involvement will likely make a significant contribution to your child's recovery.

PRINCIPLES FOR PLAYING A SUPPORTING ROLE

In the following pages, we discuss how you might be involved in intensive treatments (such as inpatient programs, residential programs, and day programs), as well as in outpatient psychotherapies, especially individual approaches. Your involvement in any of these forms of treatment will vary in the particulars, but there are some general principles that apply to all of them.

1. Agree on the Approach You Will Try

As we've stressed from the outset, one of the biggest obstacles to helping your child recover is disagreement between parents about how to help. How you can address these difficulties is detailed in Chapter 9. However, even before you make the first appointment, try to get your heads together to see if you can determine where the differences are and identify the treatment that makes the most sense for your child and family.

Chapter 6 gives information on the data available on the effectiveness of each type of therapy. If you don't find the therapy you're considering in that chapter, ask the referring doctor why he believes that type of treatment may help and why it might be a better choice than the therapies that show the greatest effectiveness in recent, reliable research. If the doctor does not have an answer that satisfies you, and the therapy does not fall into any of the categories discussed in Chapter 6, you can be fairly sure that there is no reason to expect it to be effective in improving your child's symptoms, which means that wasting time on it could endanger your child's health needlessly. Ask for another referral, and if you don't get one, see the Resources section of this book for other ideas on finding a good source of help.

When we advise you to come to agreement on which approach to try, we mean that you should include only you and your child's other parent or guardian. Don't make your child part of this decision. It's counterproductive to allow your child to have too much say in which steps will be taken to eliminate an eating disorder because, before your child begins to recover, when you talk to her about the problem, you'll end up hearing from the disorder more than from your daughter. This doesn't mean that you cannot ask for your child's opinions, but the decision remains in your hands as parents. By reading this book, you are preparing yourself to make a decision on how to help your child with an eating disorder. Your child may have opinions and strong feelings about what treatment is desirable, but as you now know, motivation for recovery is not high in many children and adolescents with eating disorders. Ultimately, then, it will be up to you to assess the treatment options and to decide how best to proceed.

2. Learn All You Can about Any Treatment You Choose

The introduction to the various treatment approaches for eating disorders we provide in this book is limited in scope and detail. So, as you consider the different options in more detail, you should seek out additional resources and information. Chapter 6 contains information on research evidence as of the publication of this book, but data from ongoing studies are always accumulating, so you may want to stay abreast of any results published in the interim. The Resources and Further Reading sections of this book will give you sources to consult for both types of information. Your child's pediatrician, too, may be able to tell you where you'll find reliable sources of up-to-date research, and if you are already working with a therapist, she may be able to provide you with handouts about various treatment approaches.

3. Share Your Perspectives on Your Child and the Child's Treatment from the Start

As we've said, anyone who is treating your child should ask you to describe your child's development and to give your observations of the child's current behaviors and symptoms. However, you should also take the opportunity to share as much as you can about what you think are contributing problems and conflicts, as well as any strengths and abilities that may be called on in both your child and your family as a whole. Providing this information and sharing your perspectives with your therapist will allow you to begin to forge a relationship in which you are working together from the start. If you have trouble in continuing to work together, Chapter 10 has ideas for improving your teamwork.

4. Keep in Frequent Contact with Any Therapists or Physicians Involved in Providing Treatment

Sometimes parents feel that once a professional is involved, their responsibility is over. Other parents feel they cannot or should not ask a therapist questions or get feedback on how their child is doing. Neither of these is a sound perspective. Although there are some areas in which confidentiality between a teenager and his individual therapist should and must be respected (sexual behaviors, intimate feelings, social activities), you still need to be involved. Regardless of the approach, your perspectives on why the disorder developed, how symptoms are currently being expressed, and how you and your family are being affected by your teen's ongoing struggles are all appropriate areas for regular discussions with the therapist.

5. Determine How You Will Assess Progress

One thing that is helpful to ask the therapist at the beginning of treatment is what to expect in terms of improvement of symptoms and over what time period. This way everyone has an agreed-upon benchmark to use that, though not ironclad, will likely help everyone see the trajectory of recovery. If you also agree on how and when you'll be updated on how things are going, you'll go a long way toward ensuring that your child is getting the treatment needed at this time. This updating should be negotiated between you, the therapist, and your child to allow you to evaluate how things are going at reasonable intervals. For example, with a teen who suffers from anorexia, never knowing for sure whether your child is gaining weight will make it difficult for you to assess your child's progress.

Also, if your child purges, but does so surreptitiously, you might not know when she's doing better or worse.

6. Have a Backup Plan

Although one of the biggest mistakes we see parents make is to keep changing therapists and treatment approaches, we nonetheless feel that you should keep your options open in case the approach you take doesn't work for your child. No treatment for any condition works 100% of the time for everyone, so it's best to be prepared with an alternate plan should progress not be as you, your child, and the therapist had hoped. Having a backup plan is not the same as undercutting a current therapy, but rather a way of making sure you aren't caught without alternatives—because, as we've said many times throughout this book, the longer these problems persist, the harder they are to change. To make a backup plan, work together as parents with your therapist and physician to see what would be the best next step as soon as progress is definitively stalled. The treatments described in Chapter 6 should provide a good start for you in evaluating your options.

7. Keep Your Child in Treatment

Although your role in most forms of individual therapy is somewhat circumscribed, it's still very important, partly because your child's motivation to be treated for eating problems is initially apt to be low. So you can expect that you will need to encourage, support, and even insist on your adolescent's attending treatment sessions. This may mean that you will have to work with your child's school to excuse him from classes so he can attend treatment, inasmuch as it is usually impossible for all therapy sessions to take place outside of school hours. This issue can cause another struggle with your child, who may not want to miss classes or time with friends. In addition, you will likely be asked to participate in some treatment sessions. The content of these sessions will vary, depending on the type of therapy your child is being provided. Regardless, make it a priority to attend these sessions. Your attendance helps send a message that you support the treatment even if you're not the main player.

HOW YOU CAN STAY INVOLVED EVEN WHEN YOU'RE NOT IN CHARGE

Throughout this book we have acknowledged how difficult it can be to be excluded from your child's treatment, whether you're just left uninformed or told directly to stay out of it. It's especially tough when this catches you off guard. If you don't know how you *can* participate, you'll feel pretty powerless to find a role in your child's recovery. The rest of this chapter illustrates specific ways you can remain involved in various forms of therapy. Even though inpatient treatment is neither the most common nor the best-studied treatment setting, it serves as a paradigm for parental participation when you're not directly in charge of treatment, as you would be in FBT, so we'll start there.

What is your role in intensive treatments (hospitals, residential programs, and day-treatment programs)?

Unfortunately, many children with eating disorders need intensive treatment provided in some type of institutional setting. Depending on the goals of these programs, the term of inpatient treatment may range from just a few days up to 12 weeks or longer. When inpatient treatment is used purely to stabilize an adolescent's acute medical problems, such as when the patient needs rehydration, the stay will likely be only a few days long and probably in a pediatric medical unit rather than an eating disorders unit. When the primary goal for inpatient treatment is to restore weight and change behaviors and attitudes, inpatient treatment might last much longer. However, for some programs the main treatment goal is simply to halt rapid weight loss and jump-start weight restoration. In these instances, rather than providing several weeks of treatment, the stay might be only 10–14 days.

What you should take from this information is that you need to be sure inpatient treatment is recommended at the right time and for the right reasons. Too often, we meet parents who have felt pressured to admit their child when they were not considered in the decision-making process. Specifically, they did not receive an adequate

Playing a Supporting Role

explanation of the necessity for this particular course of action, the goals of the admission, the anticipated length of hospitalization, and why an outpatient treatment was not considered. At other times, the converse is true, when there is pressure to keep patients out of the hospital when it is, in fact, required. Instead, the child is kept in inadequate outpatient treatment because of costs. Some parents, with the help of their doctors and considerable amounts of lobbying, have succeeded in convincing their insurance companies of the dire need for hospitalization. This route, however, is not only frustrating but also very time-consuming, especially when inpatient care is urgently required. It is best to discuss your options with your child's doctor when you are concerned about your child's weight loss.

The criteria used to recommend that your child be admitted for an eating disorder will vary from one inpatient treatment team to another, but the differences should be in nuance as opposed to substance. Both you and your child's treatment team should generally adhere to most of the following guidelines when deciding whether your child should become an inpatient for acute medical reasons (a couple of days in the case of rehydration, for instance) or for a longer-term admission for weight restoration (several weeks, as discussed earlier). General guidelines for medical hospitalization for malnutrition in adolescents have been published by the Society for Adolescent Medicine and the American Academy of Pediatrics. The precise guidelines will have to be established by your child's pediatrician, but in general they should resemble the following:

- Severe malnutrition (less than 75% of expected body weight)
- Pulse rate less than 50 beats per minute during the day, less than 46 beats per minute at night
- Temperature less than 36.4 degrees Celsius during the day, less than 36.0 degrees Celsius at night
- Orthostatic (lying to standing) systolic blood pressure greater than 10 millimeters of mercury, or pulse change greater than 35 beats per minute
- Irregular or slow pulse
- Abnormal electrolytes (usually potassium less than 3.0 milliequivalents per liter)

It is important to note that these general guidelines are based on consensus medical opinion and have not been rigorously tested scientifically: Some physicians do not necessarily agree with them. Furthermore, these guidelines address the effects of rapid weight loss, malnutrition, and purging behaviors primarily in the adolescent age group. However, younger children and adults, and persons with avoidant/restrictive food intake disorder (ARFID) can also become seriously medically compromised, and some hospitals may then apply these guidelines.

The need for a child to be hospitalized almost always causes considerable worry. Parents often approach inpatient treatment with just about as much trepidation as their child. Their uncertainty is further increased because the child, wanting to stay out of the hospital, exerts pressure on them. Although parent and child may have different reasons for feeling ambivalent about inpatient treatment, it's important to keep in mind that hospitalization reflects a crisis and is therefore often experienced as traumatic and certainly disruptive.

The only way to limit the impact of hospitalization is to keep the hospitalization brief, but this decision may be entirely out of your hands. So, taking your child for inpatient treatment is no easy decision. However, even if your child is in need of longer-term inpatient treatment, but it is possible to have her admitted for only a short stay, this could be a life-saving step you might have to take.

When you're weighing the possible effectiveness of inpatient treatment for your child against that of other treatment modes, be sure to consider what kind of follow-up treatment to the inpatient stay will be available. Without proper follow-up, it's often very difficult to maintain the improvements that have been achieved while the child was an inpatient. If the specialist unit at which your child may become an inpatient is near your home, regular follow-up appointments with your child's doctors may not be very complicated. If the facility is not close by, however, is another source of follow-up care on an outpatient or day-patient basis accessible? Making sure that your child's inpatient care is complemented by good follow-up treatment should be a combined effort between you and the discharging inpatient team. Make sure the team is willing and able to help in this way before making a decision on inpatient care.

Yet perhaps the most important issue at stake is your involvement in your child's inpatient treatment. How much and in what ways you're permitted to be involved while your child is an inpatient will vary with the treatment approach taken by the team, but it's important that you avail yourself of every opportunity offered to you. This is another reason that location is important. If the specialist unit at which your child will be an inpatient is far away, participating day by day may be logistically difficult for you. Yet this participation will help lay the groundwork for you to be active in maintaining your child's gains during the follow-up period after discharge. We have already alluded to the fact that many teenagers end up returning to the hospital because they don't sustain the weight gains they made during their hospitalizations, as Brenda's case illustrates.

> Brenda was only 12 when she was first admitted to a very well-known inpatient unit a couple of states away from where her family lived. There was no such facility within Brenda's home state. She progressed well in the hospital and was sent home after several weeks to "take care" of her eating by herself. Unfortunately, her parents, bewildered on the sidelines and against their own better judgment, watched Brenda promptly lose weight, and they had to make the trip across state lines once again. As with the first admission, Brenda settled down in the unit and started gaining weight. Her parents were not involved in the hospital's refeeding efforts and weren't given much feedback about how they might be able to help Brenda once she was discharged again. As before, with the encouragement of the nursing staff, Brenda did really well in terms of her eating. She was discharged after several weeks at a healthy weight, and again her parents were told that it was now "up to Brenda to take care of herself." Thirteen-year-old Brenda tried hard to cope with her anxieties about eating, but again her parents remained on the sidelines as they were instructed. Consequently, she lost all the weight she had gained in the hospital just a few weeks after returning home. By now, Brenda's parents knew the road to the inpatient unit all too well. The same scenario was repeated once more.

Obviously, everyone interested in Brenda's well-being would have liked to prevent this type of cycle. To avoid the same trap with your own child, we encourage you to learn as much as you can from the inpatient team while your child is there. Here are the kinds of opportunities to look for:

1. **Parent education meetings:** These meetings are common in most inpatient settings. They provide you with an opportunity to ask questions about anorexia and bulimia and to learn more about these illnesses from experts, who will also have some specific knowledge about your child and the situation.

2. **Observation of nursing and other professional staff:** If you observe experienced staff members doing their jobs, you may learn why and how they are successful at getting your child to eat and gain weight when you haven't been. You will likely notice that they don't argue about what should be eaten or when—these expectations are clearly established.

3. **Opportunities to try helping your child eat while she's in the hospital:** Some programs encourage parents to come in for some meals to allow them to see what their child is eating and to allow them to attempt to monitor a meal themselves.

4. **Discussions with the nutritionist:** A meeting with a nutritionist while your child is in the hospital can be helpful. A nutritionist can help you understand better how much food and what types might be most helpful for your child.

5. **Parent support groups and therapy:** Many inpatient programs have support groups for parents. These groups will help you see that your struggles are not unique and can provide a useful tonic for the feelings of isolation and shame that are common to families when they first struggle with a child with an eating disorder.

Unfortunately, too often parents are excluded, or exclude themselves, from inpatient programs. This can result in a cycle of weight gain in the inpatient setting, followed by rapid weight loss at home. Eventually the patient is "blamed" for not wanting to change, the parents' skills are not capitalized on, and the result is that the teenager is sent away to spend several months at a residential facility, which is often hundreds of miles from her family and friends.

In addition to short-stay admissions, intensive day-treatment programs may be an effective alternative to longer-term, intensive inpatient treatment for some patients with eating disorders. Day treatment is sometimes recommended for those patients who have completed intensive inpatient treatment; they then "graduate" to this step-down treatment prior to being discharged from the hospital altogether. Sometimes day treatment will be deemed appropriate for a patient without the patient's having spent time in an inpatient facility. This poses a difficult decision, for essentially the doctors are telling you and your child that she is very sick but not "sick enough" to spend 24 hours a day as an inpatient—a fine line to draw.

Day treatment is sometimes a good alternative to inpatient treatment in that there is a little less disruption of regular family life and it is easier for parents to be involved in treatment. For instance, parents get to oversee an evening snack as well as all meals on the weekend. If the day program can really involve parents in the treatment, this is a good way in which parents and program staff can learn from each other, so that by the time the teen graduates from the day program, his parents are more confident that they can continue to help their child, independent of the institution.

A limitation of many residential and some inpatient and day programs is that they often do not treat younger patients (under age 14) or boys. In some instances, rightly or wrongly, residential treatment is considered a treatment of last resort. When a young person has spent a great deal of time in outpatient treatment, and may also have had several stays in an inpatient facility, and yet their illness has not responded to these treatment efforts, residential treatment is often recommended. This is not to say that every patient at such a facility has failed at prior treatments; for many patients, residential treatment is the first type of program in which they participate. But it's fair to say that, as a rule, several other treatment options are explored before most doctors (or parents, for that matter) consider residential treatment. At many residential centers a program for educating parents and parent support groups are part of the overall treatment. However, by necessity, because of distance and the cost of travel, both the scope and scale of these programs are limited. Nonetheless, if your child does need to be treated in a residential facility, try to find one that involves you as much as possible and that can provide help for you when your child is discharged home.

What is your role in general family therapy for eating disorders?

FBT does not focus on general family problems or processes; instead, the main focus is on how the family can help change specific symptoms of anorexia nervosa, bulimia nervosa, binge-eating disorder, or ARFID. In contrast, many therapists use other forms of family therapy that do not directly and specifically focus on your changing or managing your child's eating disorder symptoms. Instead, these types of family therapy try to address more general family problems and processes because they believe that these general issues contribute to either the development or maintenance of an eating disorder. As we pointed out in Chapter 6 and elsewhere, the evidence that this idea is valid is very limited, but this type of family treatment is both common and considered effective by many clinicians, so you may encounter it among the options available to your child.

In these forms of family therapy, the therapist tries to change a variety of general family processes. Specifically, the therapist wishes to identify and correct inappropriate alliances within the family, communication problems, avoidance of conflict, and suppression of individuation and separation among family members, particularly the adolescent with an eating disorder. When family therapists discuss "inappropriate alliances," what they mean is that from their perspective families work best when parents work together and have clear authority. Sometimes, though, a child may end up getting closer to one of the parents than the other. This kind of alliance can happen, for example, when a child is very ill, requiring a parent to focus almost all their energy on the child. Such an alliance can also be encouraged if there are significant problems between the parents themselves. Regardless of their origin, these alliances can interfere with parents working together, especially in terms of getting rid of an eating disorder. A therapist will attempt to help a family redress the problems created by such alliances by first identifying them and

Playing a Supporting Role

then illustrating how they are interfering with the parents' working together.

Family therapists address "communication problems" by opening the lines of dialogue. Unfortunately, many family members lose the capacity even to talk to one another. This can result from many factors, among the most common of which are parental preoccupation with work or responsibilities, parental anxiety or depression, and marital discord. A specific form of communication problem is *avoidance of conflict*. This goes beyond the general problems of communication to a reluctance to take on significant problems in order to "keep the peace" and "avoid fighting." Avoidance of conflict is held as a higher good than solving the problem. Avoiding conflict can, unfortunately, backfire and allow problems such as eating disorders to fester and grow. Therapists help families determine when and how and sometimes why they prefer to avoid conflict over approaching a problem directly even if it means a period of hostility.

Finally, some families appear to struggle with supporting the evolution of their child's independence during adolescence. Because of worry about what might happen to their child or what the family would be like if their child were more independent, some families appear to send a covert, and sometimes overt, message that they don't support their child's growing up and leaving the family. Addressing this problem means that families have to explore why it might be hard to have a family member grow up and leave them. Common reasons that have been identified by family therapists include fear that without the child present the family will disintegrate, that parents will be lonely, and an unrealistic fear that the child is too immature to leave home.

Your role in these forms of family treatment is to make yourself as open and available as possible to the examination of the kinds of problems discussed here. This may be easier said than done. It's challenging for all of us to open ourselves up to this kind of scrutiny. In addition, remember the principles offered at the beginning of this chapter: Make sure you understand how progress will be measured and that you have a backup plan in case you can honestly say that you've given the treatment a chance and are not satisfied that it's helping—or, always, if you see your child continue to lose weight or suffer other debilitating medical consequences of the eating disorder.

What is your role in individual psychodynamic approaches?

Clearly, the main argument of this book is that parents need to actively take charge of helping their children with eating disorders. We have stressed repeatedly that eating disorders distort thinking and behavior to such a degree that, as a parent, you are your child's best hope for making significant progress. Nonetheless, other approaches based on psychodynamic therapy have been shown to be helpful in addressing the developmental and emotional problems associated with eating disorders, even if not in addressing the behaviors themselves. In this way they share some similarities with the general family treatments we just discussed. Many clinicians have practiced these types of therapy for years with a sense of clinical success. There are many individual schools of thought that can loosely be grouped as psychodynamic, but adolescent-focused therapy (AFT) has been shown to be effective in treating anorexia nervosa in adolescents (see Chapter 6). We'll use it in our example of how you can be involved in individual psychodynamic psychotherapy. AFT grew out of ideas derived from a type of psychodynamic theory called *self psychology*. AFT is a psychodynamic therapy that tries to resolve developmental problems to leave the child with a strong sense of self and sustained feelings of confidence and efficacy. As it pertains to anorexia nervosa, the theory suggests that children with this disorder have difficulty with feeling assertive and independent and, as a result, confuse control over eating and weight with other psychological and emotional needs related to independence and confidence. As such, it uses the therapeutic relationship with the individual therapist as the primary vehicle for promoting change.

According to this therapeutic approach, anorexia nervosa is a self-destructive attempt to manage problems with emotional immaturity, fear, anxiety, and depression by restrictive dieting and weight loss. To find alternatives to the self-destructive strategies associated

Playing a Supporting Role

with severe dieting, patients must first learn to identify and define their emotions, both positive and negative, rather than avoid awareness of these feelings through starvation. Recovery also entails increasing their sense of effectiveness in managing problems common to adolescence, including learning to successfully separate and individuate from their family of origin. Other goals of treatment are to help the adolescent develop a healthier sense of self, her family, and the challenges of adolescence and young adulthood so that she feels stronger and more capable.

Even though the main focus of AFT is on the child, parents are routinely involved. At the beginning of AFT, parents are oriented to the rationale for and nature of this form of therapy. Therapists meet with parents in separate (collateral) meetings where they try to assess parental functioning and family dynamics and begin to provide parents with information on how they can help their child manage the developmental challenges that are affecting their child's anorexia nervosa. The therapist should explain that these sessions are designed to support the parents. Parents are educated about separation and individuation being a part of normal adolescent developmental processes and are helped to better understand that what might be regarded as normal and desirable (perfectionism, compliance) are, from the theoretical perspective of AFT, likely part of the underlying pathology of anorexia nervosa. Parents are told that improvement may lead to increasing noncompliance and disagreements with them, as testing limits in these ways is seen as normal in the quest for greater appropriate autonomy during adolescence. At the same time, a young person's withdrawal may seem problematic to some parents, but the therapist helps them understand that during the course of recovery, this should be expected because it too is normal adolescent behavior.

Over the course of AFT, the therapist will meet with you to assess the degree to which you are handling your child's difficulties appropriately and offer suggestions accordingly. This may be especially necessary for the welfare of younger or less assertive patients. In addition, you will be asked about how you are handling stresses in your child's life and respecting her need for confidentiality; again, the therapist may offer suggestions to help you in these tasks. For example, the therapist can help you limit the number of extracurricular activities or tutors the child has if the child feels that either is a problem. In short, the therapist serves as your child's advocate in these collateral sessions.

To help you appreciate your child's underlying dilemmas, the therapist will try to help you by suggesting ways to understand your child's behavior and thought processes (especially as they relate to the etiology and maintenance of anorexia nervosa) without violating the confidential trust between the therapist and your child. In this regard, it's sometimes helpful for the therapist to ask you for more information about any significant life events that your child has disclosed. The therapist will explain to your child the value of sharing this information. For example, it may provide an opportunity for parents to help or to create a better support system for the child. Moreover, in the process of talking with you, the therapist may discover information (for example, that there is severe marital discord or that one parent has an eating disorder) that, with your permission, will be useful to take back to individual therapy with your child. The therapist's conveying this information may help your child take your limitations less personally and feel less devastated by them. This may be particularly the case with adolescents who are especially self-critical and who have trouble viewing their parents as imperfect.

Thus, with AFT, your role is fundamentally to support the individual therapy designed to enhance your child's capacities for mastering her dilemmas with regard to adolescence and eating. However, as you can see, you are important in the process because you provide information, support the treatment, and open yourself to changing your own attitudes and beliefs if they interfere with your child's needs.

> Sixteen-year-old Bella had been seeing her therapist in individual treatment, and she had gradually gained weight and stopped binge eating, though she still occasionally purged when she felt she went off her diet. However, she was increasingly surly with her mother and steadfastly ignored her father whenever he spoke to her. Bella and her therapist discussed these issues and framed them as having to do with Bella's wish that her parents would treat her more like her 18-year-old brother.

The therapist asked to meet with Bella's parents to discuss their view of adolescence. Bella's mother felt that Bella was struggling with her because they were too much alike. Bella's father felt that Bella was angry because they placed restrictions on whom she could date (no one older than 17) and she had a curfew (no later than 10:00 P.M. on Fridays and Saturdays and no going out on school nights).

The therapist served as an educator and advocate for Bella in the meeting with Bella's parents. She strove to help them understand the importance of allowing some risk taking (without going overboard) to help Bella develop more confidence in her own judgment and ability to make appropriate choices. Specifically, they agreed to allow Bella a trial period of dating whom she chose as long as they could meet him and to allow her to be in charge of her curfew as long as she behaved responsibly.

After several weeks, the parents were asked to return to see how things were going. Although there had been some missteps (on one occasion Bella had stayed out very late without calling), overall her parents felt that Bella had demonstrated to them that she was capable of being more responsible than they had expected. Furthermore, the conflicts they had been experiencing had diminished. Over time, Bella gave up purging on a regular basis. Her conflicts with her parents were fewer and, gradually, she was less preoccupied with her weight as she became interested in her plans for college.

What is your role in supporting cognitive-behavioral therapy for bulimia and binge-eating disorder?

Although cognitive-behavioral therapy (CBT) for bulimia nervosa, binge-eating disorder, and ARFID is primarily a treatment involving your child and her therapist, it is reasonable and appropriate to be involved in this treatment as well. That is, you can help improve motivation, support the attempts by the therapist and your child to change behaviors and thinking, and in many cases (though not all) be involved in meal planning and monitoring for and assisting with efforts to decrease binge-eating and purging episodes. Your involvement in CBT for your child's eating disorder capitalizes on your abilities to alter your home environment to support a change in binge eating and purging, similar to what you may do in family treatment, as described in Chapter 7. However, as CBT is primarily an individual therapy, your role is somewhat different and is further delineated by the various stages of CBT.

At the start of CBT treatment, your child's therapist should explain the CBT behavioral and maintenance model of eating disorders and how the specific interventions (for example, self-monitoring, behavioral experiments, problem solving, and cognitive restructuring) are helpful treatments. This helps you understand what your child will be doing and may help you determine how you can be helpful. The first task in the first stage of CBT is typically to regularize the eating pattern to prevent binge-eating episodes for bulimia nervosa and binge-eating disorders, whereas for ARFID it may focus specifically on ways to increase the range and amount of foods regularly eaten.

> Sixteen-year-old Tanika's pattern of eating was to restrict her intake all morning and through the early afternoon. Then, when she got home from school, she would begin to eat a snack, but this quickly escalated into a binge-eating episode, followed by purging. The therapist discussed with Tanika various strategies for changing her eating pattern. The one that appealed to her most was to ask her mother to eat breakfast with her and to be home after school so that she could help her avoid binge eating. This meant that her mother had to leave work early for several weeks, but her support helped change Tanika's eating patterns enough that, after several weeks, binge eating was reduced significantly.

Self-monitoring by keeping records of foods consumed and weight is a key component of CBT, although it is sometimes challenging for adolescents because it involves both the ability to self-observe and the effort of writing down these observations. Because children are typically less skillful at self-monitoring than adults, you can support your child's efforts in CBT by helping her understand the importance of completing the food records. This may mean something as simple as asking if your child has a food log sheet on her cell phone or just gently reminding her to complete it. These records are usually

Playing a Supporting Role

private entries that your child makes to discuss with her therapist, but sometimes, especially with younger adolescents, it may be helpful to ask if you can help the child complete these records, at least at first. Moreover, parents sometimes keep logs of their own observations of their child's behaviors and apparent emotional states. These can be used as comparison documents for discussion with the therapist and adolescent as well. In addition, cell phone apps for self-monitoring are being developed. These applications can be appealing to tech-savvy adolescents and may improve self-monitoring compliance.

> Maureen was a 14-year-old with bulimia nervosa who repeatedly denied she engaged in binge eating or purging. However, the therapist routinely checked with Maureen's parents about her behaviors, and they reported that although she had had a period without binge eating, they had once again noticed a large amount of food missing and evidence in the bathrooms that purging had resumed. The therapist asked the parents to join Maureen in a session. In this session, the therapist asked the parents to share their observations and concerns. The session was not confrontational, but aimed instead at helping Maureen see that although she was minimizing her symptoms, they were still a significant problem. Maureen's mother described discovering that several boxes of cookies and pints of ice cream were missing, with no explanation for their disappearance, but said she was worried that they were too tempting for Maureen to resist. Her father, who did the cleaning in the house, reported finding evidence that Maureen had recently been throwing up in the guest bathroom and wondered how he could help her. Maureen was initially tearful and angry that her parents had "snooped" on her. However, she eventually acknowledged that it was true that she was again struggling with binge eating and purging. Her parents were not critical of her and said they understood how difficult it was to stop these behaviors. They asked what more they could do to help. Maureen and her therapist decided to meet independently of Maureen's parents to come up with some suggestions to consider.

A primary aim of the second stage of CBT for bulimia nervosa and binge-eating disorder is to continue to monitor your child and if necessary to extend progress toward or maintenance of a regular pattern of eating. The next aim is to help your child delineate the nature of feared and avoided foods and to gradually reintroduce, often with your help, some of these foods into her diet. You can be helpful in these activities by contributing your own observations of your child's behaviors. For example, a feared food—one that is likely to induce binge eating—may be ice cream. You can volunteer to go with your child to get ice cream so that you can be available to support him in eating only one cone and to help him by discussing how he feels about this challenge.

You will probably not be directly involved in the specific activities of problem solving or cognitive restructuring, wherein your child tries to identify strategies to prevent binge eating and purging, as well as problems in her thoughts and beliefs about food and weight. However, you may be a part of some of the solutions that your child and her therapist devise. For example, your child may decide that she has a problem with binge eating when she's alone after school. You may be asked to be available during that time to help prevent binge eating. Or your child's beliefs about attractiveness may overemphasize weight as a focus, in which case you can provide insight and assistance in thinking about these issues in the context of your family.

The final stage of CBT is concerned primarily with the maintenance of improvement following treatment. Progress is reviewed, and realistic expectations are established. Relapse-prevention strategies are used to prepare for future setbacks. You can be helpful by identifying upcoming situations that may be stressful and by establishing yourself as a resource for your adolescent to turn to if things become difficult again. Your involvement in CBT helps acknowledge the illness and ultimately reduce shame in your child, so that help (and particularly your help), should it be needed, can be asked for sooner rather than later.

CBT for ARFID recommends that parents of children under about 12 years of age be highly involved in behavioral management strategies to increase consumption of an appropriate amount and range of foods. Older children, adolescents, and young adults usually manage these changes independently of parents for the most part. However, it is still important that information about progress,

Playing a Supporting Role

challenges, and ways you might be helpful be part of the overall treatment process.

What is your role in interpersonal psychotherapy for bulimia and binge-eating disorder?

Although adults treated with interpersonal psychotherapy (IPT) are often seen alone, therapists who treat adolescents using this approach would generally include you in the treatment because you play such an important role in the interpersonal dilemmas of your child. Remember that IPT approaches changing disordered eating behaviors related to bulimia nervosa very indirectly. However, IPT is still a very focused treatment, and your importance to the specific tasks is highlighted in the examples that follow.

As is the case with CBT, motivation of the child to attend sessions may be the initial point of entry for parents:

> Sixteen-year-old Felicity eagerly began treatment for bulimia nervosa because she was interested in working on her problems with friends. However, Felicity tended to either forget appointments or show up half an hour late. The therapist discussed how she could improve Felicity's attendance and suggested that her parents could remind her when sessions were scheduled by calling her on her cell phone in advance. Felicity agreed that this would help. Her parents were happy to assist in Felicity's treatment, and this involvement seemed to them and to Felicity to be supportive but not intrusive. In addition, Felicity's therapist had only daytime appointments, and so it was necessary to contact Felicity's school (with Felicity's parents' permission) to ask that she be excused from classes for treatment. Contact with the school's counselor helped the school administration support treatment as well.

In IPT for adolescents there are five main problem areas: grief, role disputes, role transitions, interpersonal deficits, and single-parent families. You are likely to play a role in working on some aspect of each of these areas. The most pertinent for working with adolescents with eating disorders are role disputes, role transitions, and the impact of having only one parent.

Role disputes are differences of opinion about the readiness to take up certain adult roles or behaviors (for example, dating, jobs). Adolescents frequently act out their role disputes with parents through disruptive, antisocial, or self-punishing behaviors. What differs in helping with conflicts and role disputes with adolescents is the nature of the problem and your involvement as parents. Your child's therapist will attempt to preserve workable family relationships and to provide alternatives to the disruptive behavior. To do this, it is often useful if you come to some sessions to facilitate the negotiation of these disputes, with the therapist present to help you.

> Mandy was a 14-year-old who had recently developed bulimia nervosa. She began to skip school, was caught drinking alcohol, and on two occasions met a male friend late at night in a park. Her parents were furious at her behaviors and confused by them, as Mandy had previously been a straight-A student and model child. The therapist helped the parents and Mandy realize that Mandy was struggling to assert herself and develop a sense of independence from her mother, in particular, who tended to be controlling and intrusive (mostly out of love and interest).
>
> Nonetheless, both the therapist and Mandy's parents were worried about the seriousness of the risks that Mandy was taking. Mandy's parents were considering sending her to a residential treatment setting, where someone "could keep a better eye on her." Mandy had a good relationship with her therapist and trusted him to help her. She admitted that at times she too was worried about her behaviors and didn't really understand why she did such things. She reported that she enjoyed drinking because it took her mind off her problems but that she felt vulnerable and a bit stupid for going out late at night to a park where she might get hurt. The therapist discussed with Mandy what was happening with her parents and wondered with her if she was deliberately using these behaviors to "fight" with them. Mandy agreed that she was angry at her parents, particularly her mother, who still made her lunch and bought her clothes for her. She couldn't quite see how this made her do the things she was doing, but she did know that her relationship with her parents was stressful to her.

When the therapist invited Mandy's parents to a session, the aim was to help Mandy describe how her relationship with her parents was stressful to her and to help them think about how things might change. The therapist explained that the conflict they were having among themselves was increasing Mandy's discomfort and that she herself recognized problems with what she was doing. During the session the therapist encouraged further discussion of Mandy's anger at her mother, and Mandy expressed her wish for more age-appropriate freedoms. Her mother agreed to try expanding Mandy's freedoms, though it would be difficult for her, if Mandy also promised to refrain from drinking and sneaking out at night. This initial session was followed by several others that specifically examined the changes the parents and Mandy were making and the effects of those changes on their relationships with one another. Over the next few months, disputes and conflicts diminished, and Mandy was more responsible in terms of her risk-taking behaviors.

Both adolescents and adults experience role transitions. Normal role transitions for adolescents include passage into puberty, shift from group to dyadic relationships, initiation of sexual desires and relationships, separation from parents and family, work, college, and career planning. The strategies for addressing role transitions in adolescents do not differ significantly from those used with adults, but the therapist will often want and need you, the adolescent's parents, to be included in treatment sessions. The therapist would particularly include you to support the adolescent's giving up a role and to help the family adjust to normative role transitions.

Eighteen-year-old Tanya was preparing to leave for college when her mother discovered Tanya had bulimia. Tanya's parents were anxious for her safety while she was in college and told her that their payment of tuition was dependent on her seeking treatment. The therapist helped focus Tanya and her family on the importance of the impending role transition that would occur when she went to college. This required that the parents attend several sessions, but the major focus was on Tanya's guilt about leaving home and her anxiety about going to college. To address these issues, the therapist had to help the family acknowledge to one another that this was a significant shift in their relationships and that this change entailed a loss, in the sense that the previous relationships based on cohabitation and day-to-day meetings would be forgone. They were also asked to focus on the opportunity to forge a new relationship with one another based on a more adult way of being together. The parents said that they were worried about how Tanya would do without them. They had questions for her about how she would manage the temptations of drug and alcohol use, boyfriends, and commitment to study. Tanya, for her part, listened patiently to her parents' questions and reminded them that she had some experience with all these issues and that she had thus far managed them well. She admitted, however, to also feeling worry about what it would be like to be alone more. Tanya's parents described their own experiences of going off to college and were supportive.

Single-parent families (whether resulting from divorce, death, or parental choice) are an added interpersonal focus for adolescent IPT. Not only is the child's relationship with the absent parent affected, but also her relationship with the remaining parent. Interpersonal tasks associated with this problem area include (1) acknowledging that having a single-parent family is a problem to the adolescent; (2) addressing any feelings of loss, rejection, abandonment, and/or punishment; (3) clarifying expectations for how to relate to the absent parent; (4) negotiating a working relationship with the remaining parent; (5) establishing a relationship with the absent parent, if possible; and (6) accepting the permanence of the situation.

Fifteen-year-old April developed binge-eating disorder approximately 2 years ago when her father gained sole custody of her. Her mother suffered from a substance abuse disorder. April had not lived with her father since she was 5 years old and told her therapist that her binge-eating symptoms had worsened since living with him. The therapist helped April assess the importance of her life with her single father as it related to (1) her guilty feelings about having been abandoned by her mother, (2) her anger at her father for not being in her life previously and for failing to protect her from her mother's behaviors while she (her mother) was intoxicated, (3) her wish for a female figure with whom she could discuss her romantic relationships, and (4) her wish to reconcile her parents so they would both be available to her.

Playing a Supporting Role

As we've said, the treatments discussed in this chapter are focused on helping your adolescent make changes in his own behavior while you take a supporting role. In many cases, the targeted behaviors are not the eating-related behaviors that are causing your child's health to deteriorate. This means that you should be vigilant in monitoring your child's progress, as well as supportive of the efforts made in therapy. If a child with anorexia continues to lose weight, or if a child with bulimia or binge-eating disorder continues to binge eat—and especially if these behaviors worsen—you need to take action to get your child medical help quickly and put into effect the backup plan recommended at the beginning of this chapter.

What is your role in dialectical behavior therapy for bulimia and binge-eating disorder?

Dialectical behavior therapy (DBT) is designed to help adolescents with eating disorders by teaching a range of skills in emotion regulation, interpersonal effectiveness, distress tolerance, and mindfulness that are flexibly applied in contexts where dysfunctional behaviors (for example, binge eating, cutting, substance use) would be used to regulate these negative emotions. These skills can be taught in an individual or group format. In individually based DBT, therapists try to help adolescents by scaffolding skill acquisition through practice in joint sessions with parents. An alternative model for involving parents in DBT is through multifamily groups, where a group of five or six adolescents learn skills side by side with their parents. In the individual DBT model, the specific issues of an adolescent receive greater focus, while in the multifamily group adolescents and parents get support and learn from one another. In either form, DBT tries to support the emerging autonomy of adolescents in a family context.

What is your role in cognitive remediation therapy for eating disorders?

Cognitive remediation therapy (CRT) is a treatment that tries to change the style of thinking found in many patients with eating disorders. In particular, it uses cognitive exercises to improve flexibility and big-picture thinking. There is no direct focus on weight, eating, or eating-related psychopathology, and for this reason CRT is best used only in the context of more focused treatment of the eating disorder. CRT encourages the adolescent to consider how his thinking style affects other situations in his life. During the sessions, feedback focuses on skills to challenge these thinking styles and how these skills can be used and maintained outside of the sessions. The content of the sessions is tailored to the patient's progress. Sessions usually include 8–10 tasks, followed by a conversation between therapist and adolescent about their experience and thoughts about the exercise. Parents are not involved in CRT but can provide support for the child's attendance.

Only time will produce additional data to reveal which types of therapy are most effective in saving lives being damaged by eating disorders. For now, remember that you have a right and a responsibility to be involved in your child's care. In the next two chapters we turn to possible impediments to your success in finding ways to help your child, particularly if you are taking direct charge of changing behaviors.

The next chapter focuses on working together as parents and the dilemmas with seeing eye to eye on treatment choices and the management of eating-related behaviors. However, even when you overcome your own disagreements as parents, you may encounter problems in working with your treatment team. So in our final chapter we turn to the difficulties you may face in working with professionals and with staying empowered and effective as parents fighting against your child's eating disorder.

FOR MORE INFORMATION

Fairburn, C. G., A Cognitive Behavioural Approach to the Treatment of Bulimia, *Psychological Medicine*, 1981, *11*(4), 707–711.

Fairburn, C. G., Interpersonal Psychotherapy for Bulimia Nervosa, in D. M. Garner and P. E. Garfinkel, Editors, *Handbook of Treatment for Eating Disorders, Second Edition,* 1997. New York: Guilford Press, pp. 278–294.

Le Grange, D., J. Lock, and M. Dymek, Family-Based Therapy for Adolescents with Bulimia Nervosa, *American Journal of Psychotherapy,* 2003, *57,* 237–251.

Lock, J., Adjusting Cognitive Behavioral Therapy for Adolescent Bulimia Nervosa: Results of a Case Series, *American Journal of Psychotherapy,* 2005, *59,* 267–281.

Lock, J., *Adolescent-Focused Therapy for Anorexia Nervosa: A Developmental Approach,* 2020. New York: Guilford Press.

Lock, J., S. Agras, D. Le Grange, et al., Randomized Clinical Trial Comparing Family-Based Treatment to Adolescent-Focused Individual Therapy for Adolescents with Anorexia Nervosa, *Archives of General Psychiatry,* 2010, *67,* 1025–1032.

Mufson, L., K. P. Dorta, D. Moreau, and M. M. Weissman, *Interpersonal Psychotherapy for Depressed Adolescents, Second Edition,* 2004. New York: Guilford Press.

Robin, A. L., P. T. Siegel, A. W. Moye, et al., A Controlled Comparison of Family versus Individual Therapy for Adolescents with Anorexia Nervosa, *Journal of the American Academy of Child and Adolescent Psychiatry,* 1999, *38*(12), 1482–1489.

Safer, D., J. Couturier, and J. Lock, Dialectical Behavior Therapy Modified for Adolescent Binge Eating Disorders: A Case Report, *Cognitive and Behavioral Practice,* 2007, *14,* 157–167.

Safer, D., C. F. Telch, and E. Chen, *Dialectical Behavior Therapy for Binge Eating and Bulimia,* 2009. New York: Guilford Press.

Tanofsky-Kraff, M., D. Wilfley, J. Young, et al., A Pilot Study of Interpersonal Psychotherapy for Preventing Excess Weight Gain in Adolescent Girls At-Risk for Obesity, *International Journal of Eating Disorders,* 2010, *43,* 701–706.

CHAPTER 9

Harnessing the Power of Unity

How to Stay on the Same Page in Your Fight against Eating Disorders

This chapter focuses on the challenges that two-parent families face when trying to develop a shared approach to helping their child with an eating disorder. We recognize that families come in many forms and that not all families have two parents. However, this remains the most common family structure, and in many families with two parents (or two parental figures) finding agreement can be very challenging. It so important that we feel it is necessary to devote an entire chapter to this topic.

A good specialist inpatient unit often succeeds in helping children eat normally and, in the case of anorexia nervosa, gain weight in part because a nursing team is on hand 24 hours a day to tackle the problem consistently and persistently. This is what you need to do within your family unit if you're to succeed in helping your child conquer her eating disorder: Unite as a family and stay on the same page, all the time. As we've said before, the fact that children tend to relapse after hospitalization underscores the inability of many families to present the same united front. And with outpatient care being the dominant form of treatment today, it's obvious that parents (with backup from siblings wherever possible) need to learn to come to agreement on exactly how they will participate in their child's fight for health and how they'll stick with it for as long as it takes.

If your daughter has anorexia nervosa, you must figure out how you can develop a united front in getting her to eat. If your child has bulimia nervosa or binge-eating disorder, you need to find a consistent path toward helping him eat normal amounts of food (and with bulimia nervosa, not purge). For children with avoidant/restrictive food intake disorder (ARFID), when the disorder has been present for a long period and seems impossible to change, a way forward that prioritizes overcoming it is crucial. In Chapters 7 and 8 we showed you what your role might involve if your therapist is using a family approach or another type of treatment to help your child. But even if you adhere to our principles and guidelines, you'll be surprised by how quickly any positive achievements will crumble if you don't spend as much effort on building a united front.

Developing a united front may seem straightforward. You may even feel you don't need this chapter. After all, you know that you and your child's other parent are already in agreement on wanting your son or daughter to get better. Unfortunately, where there's a will, there's not necessarily a way, unless it's exactly the same way and it's well thought out in advance. Wanting to see your child get better is not the same as both of you doing exactly the same thing to make that recovery happen. You and your child's other parent must "be on the same page" regarding the urgency of the problem, when and how to pursue professional help, and what to do at home—deciding what to say to your child to get him to eat or to avoid purging, how much food is appropriate, what consequences should be established for lack of progress, how the other kids in the family should be involved, what family sacrifices will be made to facilitate change for the child, and even details such as whether the child has to drink whole milk or skim milk. And you have to stay on the same page every minute of every day.

If you're a typical couple, you may find the idea of being in such constant agreement laughably unrealistic. Most couples have disagreements, some more than others. That's not the issue here. Despite these everyday conflicts, most parents are 100% in agreement that they want their child to recover. The issue here is to figure out how you can work together so that there is no room for the eating disorder to slip through, as evidenced in many of our illustrations in Chapter 7. Only then will your efforts to help your child really bear fruit. So, resolve to set your other disagreements aside; on this life-and-death matter, you can agree to agree.

DIVIDE AND CONQUER: HOW EATING DISORDERS SLIP THROUGH

If it's still hard for you to picture your child's eating disorder slipping through your defenses when both parents are so committed to the recovery process, imagine a fishing net. If the holes in the net are too big, the fish will just slip through. Your family, too, must be tightly woven if you're to keep your child's eating disorder from slipping through. In fact, just like a fisherman, you'll need to check the integrity of your net regularly. Holes have a way of appearing where you least expect them. For instance, you may think you and your child's other parent are saying the same thing, while your child with an eating disorder hears two different messages.

> Samantha's mother, Jill, says in a strident voice, "For goodness's sake, Samantha, eat now!" Her father, Carson, rebuffs his spouse by saying, "Don't be so hard on Samantha" before turning to Samantha and saying, "Come on, Sammy dear, just one more bite." Jill and Carson believe they're on the same page—they've both told Samantha to eat. But clearly the messages are different on the receiving end. Samantha's mother is issuing a command and already sounds angry. Carson is making a request and treating his daughter with kid gloves, in addition to criticizing his wife.

In cases like this one, which are quite common, the parents are more successful at battling each other than at finding a common strategy to battle their daughter's eating disorder. While Mom and Dad are quibbling about how to get Samantha to eat more, Samantha doesn't have to eat, and the eating disorder is given time to catch its breath, so to speak, or to "slip through." The best way for these parents to get

Harnessing the Power of Unity

Samantha to eat the amount they want her to eat is for them to really get on the same page. In fact, not just on *the same page,* but *the same line, the same word,* and *the same letter.* This will enable them to speak with one voice and say exactly the same thing: "We know it's hard for you, but we want you to eat more, and we have no choice but to find a way to help you beat this eating disorder."

In the following pages we illustrate a variety of typical disagreements between parents and how you can head them off. We hope that being aware of the insidious ways in which your child's eating disorder will try to divide and conquer the two of you will help you avoid as many of them as possible and quickly resolve those you can't. These examples will also remind you, as parents, to continue to work together in forging a path toward helping your child.

If your child has only one parent, you can still gain insight from these scenarios. As we've already shown, you may be getting help from another adult—the child's grandparent or another relative, a partner who lives with you, or even a close family friend—and that person also needs to stay on the same page as you. But even if you're going it alone, you may experience ambivalence over many of the same issues, as Tammy's mother did (see Chapter 7) when she was trying to keep her daughter from purging. Her internal conflict over how much she should control her daughter gave bulimia the loophole it needed to slip through and emerge victorious in the fight for this teenager's health. So, in the following pages, when we refer to your spouse or your child's other parent, we mean to include any other adult who is helping you in this effort.

TYPICAL DIVIDE-AND-CONQUER SCENARIOS AND HOW TO AVOID THEM

1. **Only one of the child's parents is convinced that this is the time for action and that they ought to be involved in treatment.**

    Even though everyone in the family showed up for the evaluation, Mom and Dad argued in the office about whether they should be there. "I'm not sure we should do this right now," Mom said, turning to her daughter, soliciting her agreement. Dad, fuming, said, "I'm tired of pretending that nothing's wrong. When do you think it will be time for us to do something about Rachel's not eating?"

As we've stated several times, most patients do well when their illness has been recognized relatively early on and when both parents realize the need for them to become active participants in their child's recovery. Unfortunately, several factors often work against this potential scenario. Many parents end up immobilized because they feel they are blamed for having caused their child's illness. They may feel guilty and therefore think their involvement will only make things worse, or their adolescent is pleading with them not to take her for treatment because she can "handle it" on her own. In that case it's not uncommon for one parent to give in to the pleading of the teenager, to express discomfort with "pushing" her into treatment when she so clearly doesn't want to go, or to try to convince the other parent that the adolescent isn't ready yet—"she doesn't want to change." The eating disorder is quite good at spotting this kind of opportunity, where rallying the ambivalent parent is often enough to delay any meaningful action, while the adolescent continues to starve herself and the grip of the eating disorder tightens.

This scenario is even more likely to take shape when the young person has bulimia nervosa or binge-eating disorder. With anorexia nervosa, parents can see that their child looks obviously unwell. In the case of bulimia nervosa, binge-eating disorder, and even ARFID, however, it's quite likely that parents will not be aware or will only suspect that food is disappearing or that frequent bathroom trips after mealtimes have nothing to do with "freshening up" but more with their child making herself sick to continue managing her anxiety about weight gain. Unfortunately, all these different possibilities result in the same situation—the parents feel immobilized for one reason or another, the eating disorder is good at taking advantage of this gap, and the adolescent goes without helpful treatment.

If this is the case in your family, what should you do? Try to keep your child out of discussions concerning her health care as much as possible! This may seem unfair to you—after all, she's 16 and you've

Harnessing the Power of Unity

included her in almost all recent decisions involving her. Unfortunately, eating disorders impair the ability to think rationally about treatment. Inform your child of your decision, but refrain from seeking her opinion about health care measures. That is what you and your spouse should be talking about. When you two have a private moment, try to sit down to discuss the pros and cons of your child remaining untreated. It's important to be in agreement, even if this means deciding to "give it another 10 days, but at the end of that time, we will do *X, Y,* or *Z*," as opposed to continuing to disagree while your child languishes with an eating disorder.

2. One parent's denial is actively colluding with the adolescent's illness.

> Debra's parents have been told that there is little doubt that the diagnosis is anorexia nervosa. Dad almost seemed relieved: "I knew it. I was always convinced that this was the problem. We had her visit so many doctors, from the endo guys to the GI docs and back. They couldn't find a thing wrong." Mom was less comfortable with the news: "I think we should go back to Dr. A in the GI clinic. I'm not convinced her regurgitating her food is in her head; there must be something wrong with her intestinal tract. It has to be something with her stomach or such."

Realizing that their child is seriously ill is devastating for almost all parents, so a certain amount of denial is understandable. Some parents, however, find that a diagnosis of an eating disorder remains too uncomfortable to deal with even after they finally come to terms with the fact that their child is unwell. This discomfort often results from the fact that eating disorders are psychiatric diagnoses. Unfortunately, we still live in a society in which a psychiatric illness carries a certain stigma for some, and perhaps one or both parents will find the thought of their child being mentally ill intolerable. In that case it's understandable that parents might prefer to settle for a more acceptable diagnosis, such as a gastrointestinal or endocrine disorder or another medical condition. An accurate diagnosis, however, usually leads to the right treatment, which in turn provides the best opportunity for a favorable outcome. It therefore becomes a real treatment dilemma when one or both parents are unable to accept the diagnosis of an eating disorder for their adolescent.

Just as worrisome is the fact that this scenario provides the eating-disordered thinking and dysfunctional behaviors with the ideal opportunity to thrive. Earlier in this book we characterized anorexia as ego-syntonic, meaning that the sufferer will often be unable to appreciate the severity of the disorder. In fact, we've known many patients who don't think they are ill at all! Having a parent question the validity of the eating disorder diagnosis only feeds that delusion. In the case of bulimia nervosa and binge-eating disorder, the sufferer knows that binge eating and purging are abnormal but is ashamed of the behavior and often tries to hide it. For children with ARFID, one parent may recognize the behavior as being one he exhibited as a child and argue that it is normal and the child will get over it, while the other sees a malnourished child whose growth and development are stymied. A parent's denial that a problem exists, which often happens, may only make it easier for the child to keep the problem under cover. In both cases, the family is left with a stalemate. With parents sitting in opposite camps, the illness remains untreated (or the child is treated for the side effects of her eating disorder rather than the eating disorder itself), perhaps with precious time being lost while the child is dragged from one medical test to the next in a futile pursuit of some nonexistent gastrointestinal ailment.

Once again, the crucial issue here is for parents to look at the facts together and try to reach an understanding of what the next step in treatment should be. That may be difficult, though, if the child is closely aligned with one parent in such a way that this alliance opposes or excludes the other parent, as is often the case when this scenario develops. The young person is "recruited" as an active "consultant" to at least one of the parents, leaving the other parent on the outside and quite frustrated as a result.

Debra's parents need to consult one another, not their adolescent, on these particular health concerns. If you and your child's other parent find yourself mired in disagreement about what's wrong, your child's therapist should be able to help. It's not unusual for us to devote an entire therapy session to getting a parent in denial to see the light.

3. **Each parent thinks the other one is not doing enough or not doing the right thing to make sure the eating disorder is addressed.**

> Becky is not gaining weight. Her parents are beside themselves with worry. Instead of focusing on how they can succeed at helping her next time, Dad starts in on Mom: "I told you to give her whole milk. Why do you keep insisting on skim?" Mom then feels humiliated and lashes out at Dad to remind him that he isn't doing "his job": "I asked you to have Becky eat three pancakes at breakfast, but you always seem too busy to wait around till she's done. That's no good either!"

Here the parents have indeed taken action to get their adolescent into treatment and to encourage her to eat more. These parents are also heeding the clinician's call that they work as a united team to be most effective in helping combat their child's eating disorder. However, many couples have disagreements about a variety of issues, including how they should raise their children. So, instead of just being on the same page about how they will manage their daughter's illness, these parents are trying to outdo each other. Helping their child becomes yet another way in which they battle each other instead of battling the illness. Most adolescents with an eating disorder are quite astute at realizing that parents are not quite on the same page, even though they might appear to be. These parents are making it relatively easy for their adolescent to criticize one parent—"You give me all these foods that you know I don't like"—just to have the other parent join the adolescent in criticizing that parent for not trying harder or being more creative in finding different foods that the child will eat. Needless to say, the eating disorder's strategy to divide and conquer works well in this family. The next time the young person criticizes the other parent, the remaining parent joins in the criticism, and so the cycle continues.

If you find that this happens in your family, you and your spouse should remind yourselves that disagreeing in this way is not going to help your child recover from anorexia nervosa. Although you're both trying to get her to eat more (which is good and will help her gain those much-needed pounds), you won't be nearly as successful as you could be unless you can remind yourself that on the issue of how much food, when, or how, you cannot disagree with your spouse at all! Try not to disagree in front of your child. When your spouse says something about food type or amount in front of your child and you don't agree, go along with your spouse for the moment. When the two of you have some private time, discuss your differences frankly and make sure you come to an agreement about how to handle the situation when it comes up again. Always agree in front of your child!

4. One parent blames the other for being too critical of the child with an eating disorder.

> Sasha didn't gain weight this week. Her mother seems really upset and says, "I wish you'd tried harder. I just knew yesterday that there's no way you were going to be 'up' at weigh-in today, I just knew it." Sasha looks distraught, and Dad quickly jumps to her rescue: "I wish you wouldn't always focus on the negative. You know this isn't easy for Sasha!"

In some families, there is tremendous acrimony between the parents, which is a reflection of the nature of their relationship well before the onset of the eating disorder. This does not mean that these parents will not be able to help their child. But their challenge will be to find a way to agree to disagree on many other issues and work out how they are to battle their child's eating disorder as a united team. It's very easy, however, for the young person to use these circumstances of acrimony between parents to "protect" the eating disorder. If an adolescent accuses one of his parents of being horrible, bad, unreasonable, too strict, or critical, it may be easy to get the other parent to take sides by accusing the spouse of never seeing progress, of always expecting the worst, and so on. The end result is that although both parents want their adolescent to get healthy again, they constantly get caught up in three-way struggles.

If you find yourself in this dilemma, you'll have to put your marital issues aside until your child is well again. We realize this is easier said than done. Some parents in these circumstances continually remind themselves that arguments between child and parent often lead to arguments between the parents, and that's how they remain vigilant to the eating disorder trying to slip through. But if marital discord continues to get in the way of your helping with your child's eating disorder, you should consider asking the therapist to help you address some of the crucial issues that make it so hard for you two to agree.

Although it seems fairly typical for one parent to "spoil" a child more than the other, in part because of differences in parenting style (one is permissive, one is not) and maybe also because of favoritism toward one child over the others in the family, you should attempt to find a way to avoid getting into whose approach is right. Instead, agree, as a general rule, that you'll hash out the acceptable responses to your child's food refusal—what tone of voice is appropriate, what words are okay and which are not, how you will remind each other, without being accusatory, when one of you goes beyond those parameters. As we said earlier, you should at least agree not to criticize each other at all in front of your child, but talk about these things only afterward, when alone. The best way to demonstrate your united front is for one parent to say, "Sasha, I want you to eat this plate of pasta," and for the other parent to immediately respond with, "Sasha, your mother and I want you to eat this plate of pasta." In other words, parents should repeat each other's instructions and always try to reiterate that the request for further food intake comes from both of them.

5. One parent addresses the eating disorder with relative harshness, whereas the other constantly tries to soften the verbal blows of the first parent.

"Kate, you have to eat that piece of chicken on your plate," Dad says adamantly. "I hate it when you tell me what to do," Kate retorts. Then she turns to her mother and says, "Tell him not to yell at me. You know I don't like chicken. Tell him, Mom, tell him." Kate's mother knows that it's Kate's anorexia that's trying to divert her attention to quarreling with Kate's father so that the anorexia can have its way. So she doesn't "tell him" as her daughter pushes her to do. Instead, she says, "We both know you don't like chicken, honey. No one's trying to make you eat food you don't like. Maybe you can skip your meat, just this once."

In this variation on the preceding scenario, the child's eating disorder is again trying to gain a foothold by training the parents' attention on each other and away from the illness that's causing their child to waste away. Here, however, the parents seem to be on the same page, because Kate's mother is on to anorexia's tricks. But not quite. Kate's parents may be on the same page, but they're not on the same line, the same word, and the same letter, as they need to be. They may not have gotten engaged in a dispute with each other, but anorexia did win.

Kate's mother doesn't know what else she could have done. Both parents are trying very hard to get Kate to eat more healthy meals. But if Kate's mother insists that Kate eat what's in front of her, she'll have refused to protect her daughter from her father's "bullying" and will be seen as a bully herself. If she gives in to her daughter's wishes, she'll be opposing her husband's efforts to get their daughter to eat healthier quantities of food. Kate's mother chose to bargain with the eating disorder and let Kate have a compromise meal—in this case, as is typical, a salad with fat-free dressing or no dressing at all. This scenario leaves Kate satisfied, Dad frustrated with his wife *and* daughter, and Mom embattled for trying to please both her husband and *her daughter* (read *the eating disorder*). The winner, of course, is the eating disorder.

When parents disagree about how to help their child, as these two parents have, they should always discuss their differences in private. Acting out these differences in front of the adolescent at mealtimes will only serve to blow more steam into the already invigorated illness. Even though Kate's mother felt uncomfortable with how this meal was proceeding, supporting her husband's effort (demand for eating *X, Y,* or *Z*) would have kept them on the same page. Once these parents have a private moment, they should discuss what just

Harnessing the Power of Unity

happened at the table and figure out how to deal with it when this scenario presents itself again.

6. **After some progress, one parent gets nervous about the child's weight gain and begins to criticize the other parent's efforts.**

> Juanita's mom and dad did a lot of homework together, reading as much as possible about her anorexia, investigating every treatment option, and pursuing the goal of getting their child back on track with remarkable determination. The therapist had few difficulties in convincing them of what needed to be done to make sure that Juanita started eating what she needed to eat to gain the 25 pounds she had lost in the preceding 3 months. Things went well from the treatment perspective, and every week the parents would tell their therapist how they had managed, under difficult circumstances, to make decisions together about how much their child should eat. Juanita's weight responded likewise and made good progress, with a pound or so gained every week.
>
> However, as her weight started to approach a healthy level, Juanita became increasingly uncomfortable and anxious and accused her parents of feeding her too much and making her fat. Although this was not the case, Dad started undermining Mom's efforts at helping Juanita eat sufficient amounts of food at regular intervals. "I don't think she needs to eat quite that much anymore," he would say. It turns out that Dad was also getting anxious about Juanita's weight gain. Mom, in an outburst, accused Dad of being afraid that his daughter would, in fact, become overweight: "I always suspected that you wanted her to be thin. I always knew it."

Some parents appear to be able to work well together from the start, and Juanita's parents certainly began on the same page. However, Juanita's constant pleading, especially with Dad, not to make her eat eventually convinced him that perhaps they were, in fact, "making her fat." For Juanita to reach a healthy weight, Dad needed a great deal of assurance from the therapist that he and his wife were doing the "right thing."

All parents know well what to feed their child when she is starving—it's just that the eating disorder trips them up, getting them to doubt themselves. Therefore, the challenge for Juanita's parents, especially her dad, is to remind themselves and one another that they usually do know best and should follow their gut instincts, hang in there, and listen to one another when it comes to their child's health status. If unsure, they should consult with a professional and not allow their child to counsel them on her health care needs—after all, she is only 12! Juanita, on the other hand, obviously needs her parents' assurance that they are helping her, that they only want her to be healthy and happy again. They must repeat this message jointly to her as often as needed.

What happened in this family is actually quite common. The young person manages to gain weight in the beginning, as parents have put up a united front in their efforts to help their child recover. However, in many instances the young person "goes along" in the beginning, only to find himself getting very anxious at reaching a certain level in weight gain, at which point he "slams on the brakes." The parents' challenge is to continue in their efforts even beyond this point. Their task is not only complicated at this juncture, as perhaps they are tired after a long struggle, but when one parent "agrees" with the child that "perhaps this is enough weight gain," the family has a real challenge at hand. It's not uncommon for one parent to be quite anxious about the child's weight gain, as is the case for Juanita's father. In such situations, parents need to check with one another about their goals for their child. And, as with everything else in recovery, they need to agree on what weight will be acceptable. It is important to discuss such disagreements and not allow your own possible anxieties about weight gain to get the better of you.

7. Divorce or other circumstances have created a parental triangle that makes staying on the same page almost impossible.

Diane and Lou's divorce was not amicable, and the two have a hard time speaking, much less spending time together with 16-year-old John, who has anorexia nervosa. Diane is the custodial parent, but she works the 7:00–3:00 shift at a hospital an hour's drive away. So her mother, who has her own home about 5 miles away, comes over at 7:30 to make John's breakfast before he goes to school and ensure that he eats it. It's not very convenient, but John desperately needs to gain weight, and she's willing to make this sacrifice. John then has lunch on his own at school and goes to his father's house after school, where he has his afternoon snack under Dad's supervision. He then returns home for the evening and has dinner with Mom. This array of adult caregivers involved in John's eating makes coordination of their refeeding effort extremely difficult, and John's progress has been slow. "I'm sorry," his mother has said repeatedly when their therapist has expressed concern about this arrangement. "I love my son, and I'm trying to do the best I can. But I have to go to work early, and there is no way I can get time off. We're already understaffed. If I ask for a leave, I'll lose my job permanently. Yes, of course, I'm worried about John, but his dad and grandmother will just have to help out."

Everyone in this family wants to be involved in the care of the teenage boy they love, but getting all three interested parties on the same page is quite a challenge. When such family members don't necessarily talk with one another (as is the case between Mom and her ex-husband) or live in the same home, their refeeding program is vulnerable to failure no matter how well intentioned everyone is. Because there are so many loopholes in this regimen, it's very easy for the eating disorder to find an escape route and slip through. For instance, John can easily convince Grandma that he doesn't have to have "that much" for breakfast, because "Mom already gave me so much to eat for dinner last night." John does not have to have any lunch at school because there is no one to supervise him there. When he goes to his dad's for his afternoon snack, he can announce that he doesn't feel like eating much "since I had tons of food for lunch at school." In keeping with what we have tried to make clear in previous chapters, it's not that John wants to lie to his parents, but, rather, the eating disorder is being given an ideal opportunity to slip through the cracks of this very "porous" system the adults have put in place. This family system is supposed to help John restore his weight to within a normal range for his age and height.

What needs to happen here to remedy the situation? There are many differences that may have brought on the divorce between John's parents, and Mom may have issues with her own mother because her mother has had to step in to help with child care. If John stands any chance of recovering from his anorexia, these adults will have to find a way to talk with one another, set their personal differences aside, and figure out how they can work together more successfully in John's refeeding. Their therapist should be able to help them work this out.

One possible solution is for each member of this family, after the meal for which they are responsible, to report by phone to the next person in line. Grandma calls Dad and leaves a message telling him what John ate and what John's response was to eating; Dad then decides what is an appropriate snack. Dad likewise makes a call, leaving a message for Mom so she can decide how to handle dinner. That way they don't have to talk to each other in person. Moreover, a school counselor, for instance, could be assigned the task of checking up on John discreetly at lunch to see what he's eating and maybe even offer a couple of words of encouragement. In that case, Grandma could call the counselor directly or could leave a message for Mom and Mom could make the call. Then the counselor could report to Dad.

If this schedule does not work out as planned, and all parties cannot put their differences aside, they may have to return to the therapist, who can serve as a mediator to help them communicate about how best to help John. The therapist could, for instance, designate one of the three as the "point person" who is responsible for communicating with the others and keeping track of what John is eating. In John's case, it could be his mom inasmuch as she's the custodial parent and the obvious choice, or it could be the grandmother because she may find it easier to talk to both of the others than it is for them to talk to each other.

8. One parent is very effective while the other feels defeated.

> "I feel I have to do everything to help Karen get better. I know her dad agrees with me that she's really sick, but he's given up and doesn't want to fight this illness anymore. I resent that, because

I end up being the one who has to make all the milkshakes. I'm the one who sits with Karen until she has finished her meal. I'm the one who gets up early and makes her breakfast. I think she really hates me, and all the while he gets to be the good guy."

Karen's mother understands the predicament her child is in, and she is taking appropriate steps to get her child into treatment. But she can't take much satisfaction in her accomplishments, because Karen's dad is leaving his wife to feel like the "bad cop," on top of suffering the exhaustion and resentment of handling all the food preparation and meal monitoring. Mom is, in effect, battling both Karen's illness and her husband, as the illness has been able to obtain "refuge" in Dad's abdication. This is most unfortunate, for in every setup outlined here so far, one issue is the same—while frustration and despair mount in the family, the eating disorder flourishes.

One parent can be successful in refeeding the child, or making sure she doesn't binge eat or purge, as long as this parent has the emotional support and understanding of the other parent. Some couples, whether because of personality, temperament, or mere logistics, opt to have one parent do the work. However, the important prerequisites are their agreement on the fact that their child has a serious illness and their willingness to support each other, even if this support means only emotional or psychological comfort.

Every family has its own unique set of circumstances that will determine how it responds in the face of a crisis. The important point is that regardless of this set of circumstances, the parents always have to agree on the seriousness of their child's illness and always have to agree to support each other in addressing the problem. Karen's father seems to agree that his daughter has a terrible illness, but his willingness to give up on fighting it may be his way of denying the full urgency of the problem. Or maybe it's just that he really has exhausted his personal resources for fighting the illness. Like overcoming most potentially fatal or chronic illnesses, battling an eating disorder requires quite a bit of stamina on the part of the parents. That is why it's so crucial for parents to be able to put their differences aside and figure out a way to present a united front. It's all too easy for the young person with an eating disorder to spot the differences between parents and capitalize on these differences to allow the eating disorder to persevere. If the "hardworking" parent runs out of steam, there won't be another parent to provide backup.

It is therefore imperative that Karen's parents work out an agreement whereby they can be supportive of one another. Even if Karen's mother ends up doing all the hard work of refeeding, the chances are greater that she'll be able to persevere *if* she feels Dad supports her efforts in spirit if not in body. If he feels he cannot do what his wife is doing, he should verbally support his spouse and make her feel that he is 100% behind her efforts. And he should do so in his daughter's presence so that her eating disorder knows in no uncertain terms that there is no opportunity to slip through. Being the "bad cop" on top of doing all the work would leave anyone depleted.

9. Parents take turns in siding with the adolescent (the eating disorder) against the other parent.

When parents take turns in siding with their child, the eating disorder has an ally in both parents, but not at the same time. When parents are not used to working together, they may, in fact, find it a little awkward when they do agree. This may be because they aren't used to it, or they don't really want to because they are so used to taking opposing viewpoints. When they're confronted with the prospect of figuring out together how to address their child's eating disorder, they have a real dilemma on their hands. Unfortunately, as in every scenario sketched so far, it's the adolescent's eating disorder that comes out on top. Because the parents in this example cannot see eye to eye, they will instinctively oppose each other, even when there has been progress in defeating the eating disorder. How does this look in practice?

> Dad has been quite successful at working out a schedule whereby he or his wife spends time with Brittany after every meal, whether it's watching television together, reading together, or making sure she doesn't throw up the meal she just had. Dad feels quite pleased that he has been able to help Brittany not throw up every time he's spent time with her after a meal, perhaps even to Brittany's relief. Because of Mom and Dad's long-standing

Harnessing the Power of Unity

inability to work together, however, even when it might mean helping their adolescent, Mom accuses Dad of being too rigid or too strict with Brittany and says, "How can you be supervising her like that? She's not 3 years old." Dad backs off to allow Mom to take the lead in helping Brittany. He then finds himself in a position to challenge Mom about doing something wrong when it comes to Brittany's care: "I think you made her eat that rice too fast," Dad says. "That's why she wanted to purge right after the meal. I think you should give her more time."

In the preceding scenario of endless back-and-forth bickering, Brittany's eating disorder doesn't have to do too much to render her parents' efforts relatively futile. This again points to our now familiar argument: It is absolutely essential for parents to find common ground in whatever strategy they feel most comfortable with when they address their adolescent's illness. Think of a well-oiled nursing team in a specialist inpatient unit and how the success of the team members' work is attributed mostly to their ability to speak with one voice and never to second-guess each other when it comes to addressing the eating disorder. If you and your spouse disagree, don't display this division in front of your teen. Instead, go along with the spouse who took the first step at normalizing your child's eating. Only later, perhaps after a meal and when you are on your own, let your spouse know that you disagree and discuss a compromise strategy.

STAYING ON THE RIGHT PAGE

Sometimes parents are on the same page, but it's the wrong page. They're unified in their efforts and their attitudes, but because they're headed in the wrong direction, the eating disorder is going to emerge victorious.

1. **The parents are united—but in fighting their child, not the eating disorder.**

    "I don't know when to believe Jasper anymore. He tells lies all the time. He says he doesn't vomit, and then I find all the evidence in the bathroom," Jasper's mother says. "Yes, he is really difficult. He's come to be such a negative influence in our family," his dad adds.

We discussed the importance of separating the illness from the child in our description of FBT in Chapter 7. For parents to be effective in helping their child through an eating disorder, and for the young person to know that his parents and the doctors aren't fighting him, it's very helpful to see the eating disorder as something that has overtaken him. The eating disorder should be perceived as an illness that has taken over his life, something that the young person hasn't brought on himself, and something that's most certainly not within his control. Understanding an eating disorder this way helps parents in their struggle—they are not fighting their child but are battling the illness. So, when your child finds a way to hide food, dispose of food, eat an entire cake and not tell the truth about it, or get rid of the food by throwing up, you should remind yourself that he isn't a "bad" person and is not willfully trying to deceive you. Rather, the illness gets your child to do this because he is so dreadfully anxious that weight gain will result if he doesn't throw the food away or throw up after a binge.

Naturally, then, when we propose that parents need to present a united front, we mean a united front against the illness, not against their child. In the preceding brief example, Jasper's parents are indeed on the same page, but unfortunately they are united in their disapproval of their son (because *he* lies, *he* hides food, *he* throws up, and so on). In this scenario where the parents do not separate Jasper from his eating disorder, the adolescent is left vulnerable to being overtaken by an illness that controls the way he thinks about himself, his weight, and his shape, and that powerfully influences how he behaves in response to these thoughts. He also has his parents thinking that he's a bad kid for "doing all this." The more these parents fight their child, the more they'll probably feel frustrated and be convinced that "he's doing this to spite us" or keep asking themselves and each other, "Why doesn't he just snap out of it?" The young person ends up feeling alone in his predicament and will have a very hard time convincing his parents that he isn't a bad person.

Harnessing the Power of Unity

All the while, the chances are good that his symptoms will flourish, further heightening the parents' disgust with him for throwing up, for instance, and his despair for being so utterly misunderstood.

These parents' shared inability to separate the illness from their child has made it very difficult for them to help their son through this ordeal. Jasper's parents should constantly remind themselves that an eating disorder is no different from any other illness—a young person with cancer didn't choose to have the illness, nor is he responsible for feeling miserable, tired, or in pain, or for having other illness-related feelings and behaviors.

2. The parents check with the child about important health-related decisions.

> Sharon is just not gaining much weight from week to week, and her parents can't quite understand why. It turns out that Sharon is very much involved in her own treatment planning. "Yes," her mother explains, "we always ask Sharon whether she's okay with our meal plan." "It's a good thing," Dad adds, "that she has to help us make these decisions because she has to feel she's part of the process. Otherwise, she'll feel left out and won't eat anything."

In commonsense terms, these parents sound as though they're doing the right thing. Their daughter does eventually have to make the right decisions about what to eat on her own, and so it sounds smart to get her involved now. Unfortunately, she's not yet ready. These parents have been checking with their daughter regarding her views or thoughts on a variety of subjects. Giving your child an opportunity to voice her own views and develop her own ability to make important decisions or choices is part of normal development. But when an eating disorder comes along, and *only* in terms of managing the eating disorder, you may temporarily have to take back control, at least until your child is ready to be independent again in her eating patterns.

If your child is not yet an adolescent, habitually involving the child in decision making is more a matter of parenting style than of making a natural transition to the child's evolving independence.

In this case, you may temporarily have to alter your parenting style. How you will manage your child's eating disorder by changing your parenting style will be a personal decision and will depend on the unique circumstances in each family.

> Sharon's parents know that Sharon should have ice cream for dessert. After all, she is terribly underweight, she had very little of her dinner, and she needs more calories to stave off further weight loss. They both know that and agree with one another about the course of action. Still, they can't resist asking Sharon whether she wants the ice cream. This is, after all, a reasonable thing to ask any healthy adolescent, and accepting her answer if she declined would be reasonable as well.

What Sharon's parents are forgetting is that when they talk to Sharon about food, they are not talking to a daughter who has reached the level of maturity expected of a typical 15-year-old, but to anorexia nervosa. And anorexia nervosa will always answer no. Sharon—if she were well—might very well want the ice cream, but someone overtaken by the symptoms of anorexia nervosa will certainly refuse it: "It's bad for me, it'll make me fat" or "You know I don't like ice cream" are typical responses. The result is that the parents find themselves in an awkward dilemma. They may feel that the alternative to continuing to ask such questions of their daughter is to be unacceptably "mean" or disrespectful of the kind of person she has proven herself to be. "We always let her have what she wants," said Sharon's mother. "She's such a careful and thoughtful child, and we know she'll make the right decision." This may indeed be true for every aspect other than eating, and it may have been true for all aspects of Sharon's adolescence before the eating disorder overtook her thoughts and feelings about food, weight, and shape. But it's not true now, because Sharon is not the one making the decisions about food.

What should Sharon's parents do? They have to *temporarily* find a way to avoid giving Sharon much of a choice when it comes to the foods she eats. If they feel that contradicts their parenting style and they feel they *have* to introduce choices, these choices should be between chocolate and strawberry ice cream, as opposed to ice cream or no ice cream. Although our proposal may seem somewhat dogmatic, chances for the recovery of your child are accelerated when her weight goes up, when she manages to refrain from binge eating or purging her food, and when she is supported in eating the amount and range of food needed for health instead of getting stuck in an endless "eating disorder debate"—something that is best avoided.

CAN PARENTS AGREE? THEY MUST

We've presented several typical disagreements in parents' approach to an eating disorder, each time pointing out how these disagreements can hamper your child's recovery and how your child might try to steer you away from ultimately helping her with her eating dilemma by dividing your efforts or by simply distracting you from the task at hand—her recovery. In each example, we've also pointed out what to look for in your own behavior that may, in fact, complicate the steps you've already taken to help your child. Finally, we've shown specifically how you, as parents, can work together in a way that's productive for your child, even if you and your spouse have to agree to disagree for now. We hope you'll use these examples as inspiration in your efforts to find a way to agree on how to help your child, from meal to meal and from minute to minute.

FOR MORE INFORMATION

Alexander, J., and D. Le Grange, *My Kid Is Back—Empowering Parents with Family-Based Treatment for Anorexia Nervosa, Second Edition*, 2024. New York: Routledge.

Le Grange, D., and J. Lock, Editors, *Eating Disorders in Children and Adolescents: A Clinical Handbook*, 2011. New York: Guilford Press.

Le Grange, D., and J. Lock, *Treating Bulimia in Adolescents: A Family-Based Approach*, 2007. New York: Guilford Press.

Le Grange, D., J. Lock, and M. Dymek, Family-Based Therapy for

Adolescents with Bulimia Nervosa, *American Journal of Psychotherapy*, 2003, *57*, 237–251.

Lock, J., *The Oxford Handbook of Child and Adolescent Eating Disorders: Developmental Perspectives*, 2012. New York: Oxford University Press.

Lock, J., and D. Le Grange, *Treatment Manual for Anorexia Nervosa: A Family-Based Approach, Third Edition*, 2025. New York: Guilford Press.

Lock, J., A. Whyte, B. Matheson, and N. Datta, *Family-Based Treatment for Eating Disorders Piece by Piece: A Practical Guide for Parents*, 2024. New York: Routledge.

CHAPTER 10

Staying Empowered and Informed

How to Work with Professionals Who Are Trying to Help Your Child

Professionals who are trying to help your child will always have your child's best interests at heart. That does not mean, however, that you'll always find yourself in agreement with the doctors when it comes to their treatment plan for your child. You may have to struggle to see eye to eye with your child's pediatrician, psychologist, psychiatrist, or therapist because in many cases parents are still viewed more as part of the problem than as a key to the solution. So, as much as we would like to believe that you can become a full member of your child's treatment team just by being willing and able to participate, that's not yet the case in all treatment settings. Fortunately, the mindset that resists parental involvement in the care of teenagers with eating disorders is shifting as research data supporting the importance of parents' contribution continue to accumulate. Just be aware that you may have to make a greater effort to stay informed and empowered than you might expect, which is why we've devoted a chapter to suggestions for handling the dilemmas you may encounter during your child's diagnosis and treatment.

Throughout this book we've emphasized the critical need to *stay on the same page* during your child's treatment. In Chapter 9 we looked at what that demands of two parents or other adults raising a child who has an eating disorder. But the concept applies equally to everyone involved and in contact with your child while she is recovering from an eating disorder. Not only must you and your child's other parent be on the same page, the members of the treatment team should also be in full agreement with one another and with you and your child's other parent. Obviously, this condition can't be met unless you feel your treatment team is on the right course. The value of this *agreement* among all parties should not be underestimated—it is all too easy for the adults (you and the professionals) to become confused about the right course of action to pursue, while your child's treatment suffers as a result. In the last chapter we talked about how the eating disorder can exploit disagreements to derail the efforts to get your child back to health. An eating disorder can also easily find cracks in the front established by the *entire* alliance formed to help your child—both parents and all the professionals involved. In the next several pages, we detail some potential pitfalls that might make it difficult for you to agree with your child's treatment team, as well as what you can do about such a situation so that you can remain a vital part of the solution. Although it is not possible to advise you on the specific makeup of the treatment facilities or treatment teams in your area, we hope you will read this chapter in conjunction with the information provided in the Resources section that follows and that this can help you come up with a strategy that will support your efforts to help your adolescent. Finding the best treatment facility for your child will be a challenge, but we hope that having reached this point in this book will equip you with sufficient knowledge to make an informed decision and play a constructive role in your child's recovery.

In addition to the difficulties of parents that are discussed in Chapter 9, the following are common dilemmas that parents encounter, not only in trying to stay on the same page with the practitioners treating their child but also in retaining an active role in their child's recovery. Keep in mind that the central question is not whether the professionals on your child's team are dedicated to helping her get better, but whether their treatment philosophy allows you to be fully involved. If it does not, preparing yourself to stand your ground in a constructive manner will go a long way toward enabling you to play an active part in your adolescent's treatment.

A professional you've consulted says your child's problem "cannot be an eating disorder."

There are many reasons that your child's pediatrician or other doctor might make this pronouncement. If you've agonized over the decision to seek help, your child has resisted, and you're sick with worry, this conclusion may initially provide some relief. But relief can quickly turn to increased anxiety when you know that something is wrong and the doctor has left you with no explanation or course of action, especially if, like many parents, you've been doing some research on your own and are pretty well convinced that your child has an eating disorder. What do you do?

To start, consider why the doctor has reached this conclusion. Knowing this can lead you to a next step that will get you on the path to helping your child. Is it likely that this doctor is simply not very psychologically minded and would not ordinarily consider a psychiatric diagnosis? If you have prior experience with the practitioner, what does that history tell you? Has the doctor ever suggested considering psychological factors when your child has had a problem in the past? If not, and he has said something like "I've examined Caroline very carefully, and I have given this a lot of thought. Although I can't find any medical reason for her weight loss, I just don't think it is an eating disorder," obviously, you'll need to ask him why he doesn't think this is an eating disorder and what you should do now inasmuch as your child continues to resist eating or to binge eat and purge. If the doctor suggests a "wait and see" course, you'll have to make it clear that you've already waited and that you are far too concerned about your daughter's health to allow any more time to pass before taking action. This statement can be firm without being abrasive: "Doctor, I appreciate the care you've taken to consider all the medical causes of Caroline's behavior, but I'm really worried and don't know what to do. Can you refer us to someone who has experience with eating disorders so we can be sure that ruling this out is the right thing to do?"

Another possibility is that, despite his best intentions, the pediatrician you have consulted has not based his view on all the available evidence, both medical and psychological/psychiatric. Again, you can ascertain this by asking exactly what the doctor has taken into account—"Doctor, are you satisfied that you've done all the tests to rule out a medical illness that can explain my child's weight loss? We want to be sure that every angle has been considered"—and making your own judgment about how certain the doctor seems and how thorough his assessment appears to have been. Does he respond cryptically, vaguely, or defensively? If so, it may simply be an indication that he is not very comfortable in this area. In most cases, a tactful question along these lines will give the doctor an opening to admit that he's not satisfied with his own finding and will refer you to someone else who can do more.

It's also possible that the doctor has taken into account *only* what the tests and office exam can show—not the behaviors you have observed at home or that have been reported to you by your child's school. Your child's eating habits are not going to be evident in the doctor's office, so what you and others who are around your child much of the day see her doing is critical to a diagnosis of an eating disorder. If you think the doctor has not taken your reports seriously, reiterate them. Many parents benefit from bringing a written log of the behaviors they've observed (what their child has eaten and not eaten at various times during the day, what she has said about food and eating, notable changes in behavior, exercise habits, and so forth) to the doctor's office. If you haven't already done this, and the doctor can assure you that your child is in no imminent danger (see the warning signs on pages 27–28), you might offer to construct such a log for the week ahead and then meet with the doctor again.

Although making a diagnosis of an eating disorder may be straightforward for those who work with these illnesses on a daily basis, many pediatricians and other general practitioners don't have this background. If they've seen very few cases of an eating disorder, they may be somewhat cautious to make this diagnosis. If your child is between 9 and 11 years old, it will be difficult for the doctor to recognize such a disorder even if he has been dealing with adolescents with eating disorders, because certain types of eating disorders are quite rare among young children and the manifestation of the

Staying Empowered and Informed

illness in them may be atypical. Similarly, eating disorders are not as common among boys or among some ethnic minorities, and again, the pediatrician may not be inclined to consider an eating disorder as a potential diagnosis because your child is male or a member of an ethnic minority. Finally, although avoidant/restrictive food intake disorder was added to DSM-5 in 2013, many pediatricians (and unfortunately many other health and mental health practitioners) are not familiar with it and may not recognize the need for intervention.

Unfortunately, diagnoses of eating disorders are overlooked from time to time because it's simply not the first diagnosis that medical professionals will think of—or even consider—if they haven't seen these disorders before. If your instinct and your knowledge of your child tell you that she indeed has anorexia or bulimia nervosa, for instance, you should ask for a second opinion from someone such as a child and adolescent psychiatrist or a psychologist who specializes in the treatment of eating disorders. You may be hesitant if you feel intimidated by medical professionals, or you may fear that your pediatrician will somehow be offended, that you don't trust him. But once you have put your reluctance aside, getting a referral from your child's pediatrician ought to be a relatively straightforward request and procedure. Most doctors would welcome you to explore this option, for they could also learn from the outcome of such an evaluation. If it turns out that a diagnosis of an eating disorder is confirmed, then you should consult your pediatrician about how he would like to continue to be involved in your child's medical care. Most pediatricians would want to stay involved in your child's care and would probably be quite happy to consult with your child's psychologist or psychiatrist.

A professional tells you to stay out of, or on the sidelines of, your own child's treatment.

Parents can experience a variety of forms of exclusion, such as not being a part of the core assessment and planning phase of the treatment, not being made a part of the solution by meeting with their child's doctor on a regular basis to discuss the progress in treatment, or worse still, being excluded from the treatment altogether. This approach is in stark contrast to most available evidence that supports parental involvement in the treatment of an adolescent with an eating disorder, as we have stated throughout this book. It is, therefore, quite inconceivable that treatment can be successful without the parents' constructive involvement in one form or another. If you need a reminder of the research findings in favor of parental involvement, see Chapter 6.

Many professionals, however, will follow a treatment path that mostly (or only) addresses your child's concerns and worries, while attempting to keep you at bay. Some professionals may even think of many parents as "overinvolved" and "interfering" in the treatment process. It is, therefore, not uncommon to hear parents report that their child's therapist would not meet with them or even (fortunately, more rarely) take their calls. Any of these types of exclusion can be difficult to overcome.

Although there is no "one right way" for parents to be involved in their child's treatment, you should not be excluded from being a part of making these crucial decisions at the outset of treatment. If you are not to be a part of the treatment process, you should still ask the professionals about the balance between addressing the eating disorder symptoms on the one hand and exploring the "underlying issues" on the other. It should be quite acceptable to ask your child's therapist, "Can you explain your reasoning for not including us in the treatment process?" and "Can you let us know how Sandy's medical status will be monitored throughout this process, who will weigh her and how regularly, and how we can be kept informed about her progress, in psychological as well as medical terms?"

Your aim is to make sure that the dire consequences of starvation or binge eating and purging are addressed urgently and consistently. You should be allowed to question the treatment team regarding your child's progress, in terms of both the improvement in eating disorder symptoms and the role of and emphasis on psychological treatment. If the medical aspects of your child's illness are not addressed, or if you are not informed about the progress in weight gain or cessation in bulimic symptoms, you should insist on being informed in the same way an oncologist would diligently keep parents abreast of how their child's tumor was responding to treatment.

You are given advice you don't agree with.

Regardless of the exact treatment approach, parents often feel uncomfortable about the advice given by the treatment team but don't know whether they can or even have the right to disagree. You may be told that your child's eating disorder can "be treated only in an inpatient setting" or that "the medications we have prescribed are standard for adolescents with anorexia" or that "residential treatment (in another state) is really your only option." You might be surprised to know that many other parents intuitively feel uneasy about such advice but don't think they can second-guess the professional team. "Who am I to question the doctor?" is the reaction that still pops into parents' minds when they don't feel completely comfortable with professional advice; after all, most of us have been brought up to believe that the professionals "know best." Although our advice is not aimed at setting you on a collision course with your child's treatment team, or encouraging you to immediately oppose or question every decision, you should feel comfortable, as a matter of routine, about asking your child's therapist *why* course X as opposed to Y was chosen. You should feel confident in asking your child's doctor why she has decided on medication to treat your child's bulimia and why medication A was chosen as opposed to B. Many doctors want to go into detail about their decisions but are prevented from doing so simply because of time constraints. To make sure this doesn't stand in the way of your being fully informed, you can always ask if another appointment, just to talk through all the important issues, would be wise, or you may be able to set up a regular time when you and the doctor can touch base by phone.

Most important, and perhaps more difficult for you to do, you should feel that you can tell the doctor when you disagree with the chosen treatment course. You should, of course, have a good rationale for this approach after you've done your research thoroughly. How you approach this situation is crucial, as you don't want to be seen as antagonistic and you don't want to invite your doctor to react defensively. You may start by saying, "Can you help me understand why you recommend a residential treatment program as opposed to an intensive outpatient regimen?" or "I don't understand the mechanism of the medication you have recommended. Can you explain how this works and why you've chosen this particular path?" With this approach, even though your questioning might be motivated by your disagreement with the doctor's recommendation, you've phrased your disagreement as a question for clarification. This gives your child's doctor an opportunity to provide a satisfactory rationale that may help convince you, or unfortunately, may confirm that you really cannot agree with the chosen treatment path. Most important, you should be prepared to discuss your differences with your child's doctor in an atmosphere of trying *together* to find the best course of care for your child. The likelihood that treatment will be successful is usually enhanced when everyone is in agreement and can enthusiastically endorse the route of care chosen.

Incidentally, when you have doubts about the advice you're being given, be sure to examine your reasons for feeling this way. For all the reasons discussed in Chapter 5 and elsewhere, your child may try to get you to doubt the professionals. Remember, because her thinking and judgment are severely distorted as a result of her eating disorder, she will try to find ways to perpetuate it. So, when the eating disorder speaks for your child, the effort will be to convince you that the doctor who made the diagnosis was wrong and that the treatment team's attempts to curtail the symptoms are ineffective. After all, if you buy into this claim, you might withdraw your teenager from treatment, in which case the eating disorder wins! Treatment is in serious trouble when your adolescent succeeds in getting you to question the treatment and leads you to either seek "alternative" treatment or, worse still, abandon treatment altogether.

You may start out with full faith in your child's treatment team, but the cognitive distortions that mark an eating disorder can make your child very persistent in trying to undermine the treatment and the professionals providing it. So, when you find yourself experiencing growing dissatisfaction with your child's treatment, ask yourself whether you have concrete reasons for doubting its effectiveness. If not, and you realize you're being swayed by your child, gently but firmly remind him that you, as parents, are in the best position to make treatment decisions, not him—not just because your child is still under age, but mostly because the eating disorder does not allow

Staying Empowered and Informed

him to make rational health care decisions. Also, remind your adolescent that everyone (parents and professionals) must be united in fighting the illness and that it's your goal to stay that way to give your child the best possible chance at recovery.

Your child may still feel that you're fighting him and not the illness. In this case, remind yourself to separate the illness from the adolescent: You are battling the *illness,* not your *child.* This thinking will help you stay on course, even when your adolescent puts forward "logical" arguments as to why you should question the interventions prescribed by the professionals.

If, after examining the source of your doubts, you still aren't convinced that the advice you're getting is right, remember that professionals can't always back up their treatment decisions with hard data, especially considering that the research studies on eating disorders are still so sparse, but they should nevertheless attempt to provide you with the reasons behind their decisions. It is *your* child's treatment; *asking* will make you a part of the treatment effort, and *knowing* enables you to pursue a particular treatment choice with greater conviction. In fact, you might be pleasantly surprised to find that most therapists will be all too happy to take a few extra minutes and have you think with them about the chosen route for treatment.

You've been given conflicting advice.

Because there's no uniform treatment for young people with eating disorders, it's relatively common for parents to be told one thing by doctor *A* at hospital *A* and another by doctor *B* at clinic *B*. Your dilemma, of course, is "What do I do now?" You obviously want to do what's best for your child, but your job is made considerably more difficult with two opposing viewpoints from professionals. If you find yourself in this dilemma, we can only offer some guidelines about finding the right course of action. First, and as we have suggested earlier in this chapter, ask the respective professionals the following:

- How they've arrived at their particular advice
- Which guidelines they consulted as a basis for their decisions
- How many patients they have treated this way

- What the response has been
- Whether this is standard practice among other professionals in this field
- Whether there are published data to support this approach

Although this may seem unnecessary to some, think of the questions you asked when your child was fitted with her first set of braces; think of the detail the orthodontist went into in explaining *why, what,* and *when.* It's quite acceptable to follow the same approach here, even if your child's psychiatrist appears a little reluctant to engage in this kind of discussion. Remember, it's your child's life that's at stake, and you want to be assured that you are following the right course of action. Second, and again, as we've mentioned earlier, it's important for you to feel comfortable with the advice so that you can endorse the actions necessary to help return your adolescent to a healthy state. This will happen only if the doctor takes some time walking you through the decision-making process. So, trust your gut instinct when you feel this might not be the right treatment for your child, especially in the absence of research or clinical data. *Parents are usually on target!* Pursue your concerns (within reason) until you are satisfied that you can endorse a specific treatment route.

The professionals are not on the same page.

Whereas the preceding dilemma refers to your having made visits to two different clinicians about your child's eating disorder, the difficulty presented here refers to members of your child's treatment team (two professionals under the same roof) not being in sync with one another. We've already mentioned that treatment of an eating disorder is complex, and several professionals should ideally be involved in your child's care (for example, a pediatrician, a psychiatrist, and a therapist). These doctors could inadvertently confuse you and your child by providing guidance that might differ subtly at times. Possibly the most common issue that arises concerns target weight. Doctor *A* may say, "She should probably weigh somewhere in the high teens," when your daughter's weight is just over 100 pounds

Staying Empowered and Informed

at the time. Another team member (doctor *B*), in an effort to sound encouraging, may say, "We're almost there" in response to the adolescent's begging to know how much more weight she'll have to gain, as she is just over 100 pounds now. Both doctors have the same goal in sight (a healthy weight, given the patient's height and age), but your adolescent will most likely opt to hear from doctor *B*: "Just 1 or 2 more pounds." You may be confused as well and not quite sure what the "real" message is. Without having to walk on eggshells all the time, doctors who treat patients with eating disorders need to be exquisitely careful about how they phrase information on weight gain issues. Anorexia not only speaks for the adolescent when food issues arise, it also hears for her. So the girl who is told "we're almost there" not only will prefer that message to "we have another 10 pounds to go" because it allows her to delude herself that she doesn't have to gain much more weight, she may also become very upset at the implication. This vague statement of encouragement can set off an alarm—"I must have gained *so* much weight!"—and send her out of the office in tears. It's important that goals be clear and specific and that all the members of the team agree on them.

Unfortunately, you won't be in a position to control many of these kinds of occurrences. However, it's important to understand how the eating disorder gets your child to think and respond to these events and how important it is for you to be able to check with your child's doctor when these misunderstandings arise. Discussing the distress felt by a young person who is very sensitive to any news about weight gain can only further your collective efforts to speak to your child productively. Moreover, understanding this illness can help you notice when the professionals inadvertently confuse you. Your job is to let the professionals know when this happens.

Although unintentional miscommunication is, unfortunately, a common occurrence, the team members have an obligation to make sure that they "speak with one voice." You, on the other hand, should let the team know when they confuse you about their messages or treatment goals so that ultimately everyone can stay on the same page. This will, we hope, be easy enough. Go back and tell doctors *A* and *B* that you're confused, tell them why, and have them clarify the situation. This way the doctors will be reminded of their oversight and will probably try harder to prevent this from happening again. You should definitely let them know; otherwise, they'll be unaware of the confusion they've caused.

The various professionals involved are not staying in communication when your child has several psychiatric problems requiring multiple treatments.

Treatment of an eating disorder is especially complicated and often involves a couple of professionals at the same time when other psychiatric illnesses coexist with the eating disorder. Having an anxiety disorder or depression in addition to an eating disorder will further complicate your child's treatment. This is a difficult process to manage, whether the professionals who treat your child are all part of the same team at the same institution or are located at different facilities/practices and are collectively involved in your child's treatment. In either case, the treatment team's responsibility is to stay on the same page with one another, even though they represent different professions and may approach treatment from slightly different perspectives. You need to make sure that these professionals all speak to one another *and* to you, the child's parents.

> Fifteen-year-old Darlene loves ballet. She has lost so much weight over the past few months that her pediatrician recommended she not be allowed to dance while her parents are trying to help her gain weight. Darlene is also quite depressed and meets with a psychiatrist on a regular basis. The psychiatrist treats her with antidepressant medication. So far so good. However, the psychiatrist thinks it's a good idea for Darlene to continue to dance because this makes her happy and may also help with her depression. Both of these doctors are obviously recommending what they think is best for Darlene. But Darlene has latched on to what the psychiatrist had to say about her dancing, making it very hard for her parents and her pediatrician to keep her from dancing. These two doctors should have been in touch with one another first, to make sure that they were on the same page before verbalizing their treatment plan to the family.

Staying Empowered and Informed

Although you don't want to be put into the position of having to check on the team to make sure they are doing their jobs, you want to be reassured that the various professionals involved in your child's care do, in fact, share notes with one another. You will have a clear sign that this is not happening when you hear different directives from two or more members of the treatment team, as in the example of Darlene. If this is the case, you should point out to the person who is ultimately in charge of your child's care that you are confused, as you've been hearing different directives. It's the responsibility of the team leader to clarify such inconsistencies and make sure there is a united front in the battle against your child's illness. Go back to the team leader after a while and check with her to see whether the team members have conferred with one another. In that way, you can be reassured that the dilemma has been resolved—at least for now.

Also be aware that there will be times when it is up to you to decide which of two conflicting approaches you feel is best and to steer the entire team in that direction. For example, a medical team may be quite worried about the potential for bone loss and may stress weight gain above normal to ensure that bone loss doesn't occur. The psychiatric team may see this additional weight gain at that particular point as risky because it could lead to an intensified preoccupation with weight and a relapse. You may need to study these conflicts for yourselves, to a certain extent, to determine what you believe is the current priority. Similarly, a nutritionist may recommend a particular diet plan, whereas the psychiatric team may see any prescribed "diet" as leading to a preoccupation with food that increases obsessional concerns about eating. It's often up to parents to consider the pros and cons of these professional options and sometimes force the team in a single direction. When that is the case, you can ask the professional with whom you agree for advice on how to speak tactfully to the disagreeing team member(s).

Too many cooks in the kitchen?

In Chapter 9 we mentioned that you want two cooks at most in your kitchen (you and your spouse, *not* your child) while you're attempting to normalize your child's eating habits. Likewise, you also don't want too many professionals involved in your child's care. It's incredibly confusing for everyone when a treatment team tries to address every possible angle of the eating disorder at the same time (group therapy, family therapy, individual therapy, medication, refeeding, occupational therapy, exercise therapy). Such a multifaceted approach invariably involves a pediatrician to take care of the medical issues, a psychiatrist for medication management, an individual therapist for psychotherapy, a family therapist to meet with the family, a nutritionist to consult with either you or your child, and so on. There is no research evidence that this catchall strategy will necessarily provide the results you desire. In fact, it can be very confusing and taxing for your child (who may have diminished resources, given his health status), as well as for you. Our advice here is no different from that offered for every scenario described before: You should feel that you can talk to the doctor who is ultimately in charge of your child's care and ask her why another professional has been added to the team, what the rationale is for this practitioner's involvement, what the timing of this practitioner's interventions will be, and what goals this professional hopes to achieve.

The treatment team tells you they've done everything they could and can't be of further help.

There are very few, if any, circumstances in which a treatment team should give up on a young person's treatment for an eating disorder. No doubt, hearing from your doctors that they have "tried everything" will be distressing to you and will put you, as parents, in the awkward position of disagreeing with your treatment team. You will have to try to persuade them not to give up, or you may have to go ahead and look (yet again, perhaps) for a team of professionals who will make another effort to help your child in his struggle.

Remember, the outcome for many young people with an eating disorder, if they receive good treatment, is positive. The available data show that when properly treated, most children improve and many recover from their illness. Therefore, you should question the professionals if you're told that "nothing more can be done," "your child is not ready yet," or "she's not motivated to change." Young

Staying Empowered and Informed

people with eating disorders, as a rule, don't want to get better and will not want to work with you and the treatment team to overcome this illness. Perseverance is of utmost importance if treatment is to be successful. You *and* the professionals must find a way to persist if you want to help your child overcome this illness.

If worse comes to worst, and the team just can't seem to work together, or you have disagreements with the team that you can't seem to resolve after diligent efforts to do so, it may be time to make some changes. How do you know when you've reached that point? If you've truly lost your confidence in the team, and your child is getting worse or making no improvement, it's time to consider a change. Your child's welfare is the reason you sought treatment to begin with, and the effectiveness of treatment should be the priority. Remember, though, that it's hardly ever constructive to suddenly jump from one group of professionals to another, denying any team the chance to make headway with your teenager.

You are sent from pillar to post.

Not every family with a child with an eating disorder lives in a city or state where a multidisciplinary team of specialists is available to help with the child's treatment. Consequently, you may find yourself being sent from one specialist to another, and these professionals are often in another city or even in another state. You may also have been told to have your child admitted to either a residential or inpatient facility hundreds of miles away in another state. Going back and forth like this can be confusing, and you are often left not quite knowing which avenue to pursue or even which of the available options will result in the best outcome for your adolescent.

No doubt, this is a very difficult position for you to be in—either shopping around your own city or having to think of sending your 14-year-old away to another state. The important issue here is to feel comfortable with the decision that you will be making and confident that you'll be able to stick with the course you have opted for. This sense of comfort won't be possible unless you feel you have done a fair amount of homework regarding the options available and, consequently, that you've made an informed decision. It's critical that you find a facility and group of professionals that have true expertise in treating adolescents with eating disorders. The Resources section of this book can help get you started on finding such a team, but you can also rely on referrals, track records, years of experience, board certifications, and any other criteria you would normally apply to choosing the best possible health care practitioners for any problem your child has.

So, invest in the time to shop around, because when you've made your difficult decision, it's going to be important for you to show the perseverance we just referred to. As we said at the outset of this chapter, this book should help you be better informed about your child's eating disorder and the treatment options available. When you are in the position of having to shop around or having to send your child away to a treatment facility in another state, you will now feel, with some certainty, that you have taken the best available step. In addition, as we noted in Chapter 6, videoconference delivery of treatments is effective, and an increasing number of clinicians now use this modality, improving the reach of treatments beyond specialty centers.

We've pointed out several times in this book that treatment will probably be most helpful if you're involved in every step of your child's care. Sending your child away to another state for a month or more for the professionals to get her weight back on track or normalize her eating behaviors may be helpful to your child, but she will eventually return home. You will then have to figure out a way to make sure that she doesn't relapse. To do so, you need to be involved in the treatment, and you will have to find a way to communicate this to your treatment team. As we said earlier in this chapter, some professionals would like to keep you out of treatment to a large extent. Your challenge will be either to find a team that recognizes the tremendous value parents bring to treatment or to convince a team of the resources you bring that can help ensure that your child gets back on the road toward recovery. Ask the team members how they usually involve families who travel long distances in their treatment approach.

In this chapter we presented several typical challenges that parents of our patients have experienced with professionals who are trying to help their children. These dilemmas have often resulted in the parents feeling confused and disempowered. There is no doubt that such struggles can hamper your child's recovery. In each example, we have pointed out what the source of confusion between you and your child's treatment team might be. In each case, we have encouraged you to find your voice, make sure you remain informed, and remain a part of the solution. We have also pointed out specifically how you, as parents, can work together with your treatment team in a way that will be productive in your child's recovery. In the next section of this book you'll find resources for getting the best treatment for eating disorders in the United States and other countries.

FOR MORE INFORMATION

Alexander, J., and D. Le Grange, *My Kid Is Back—Empowering Parents with Family-Based Treatment for Anorexia Nervosa, Second Edition,* 2024. New York: Routledge.

Le Grange, D., and J. Lock, Editors, *Eating Disorders in Children and Adolescents: A Clinical Handbook,* 2011. New York: Guilford Press.

Le Grange, D., and J. Lock, *Treating Bulimia in Adolescents: A Family-Based Approach,* 2007. New York: Guilford Press.

Lock, J., *The Oxford Handbook of Child and Adolescent Eating Disorders: Developmental Perspectives,* 2012. New York: Oxford University Press.

Lock, J., and D. Le Grange, *Treatment Manual for Anorexia Nervosa: A Family-Based Approach, Third Edition,* 2025. New York: Guilford Press.

Lock, J., A. Whyte, B. Matheson, and N. Datta, *Family-Based Treatment for Eating Disorders Piece by Piece: A Practical Guide for Parents,* 2024. New York: Routledge.

Resources

The resources in this section are not comprehensive or exhaustive, but should provide guidance in identifying some programs and treatment centers near you. We recognize that this list is mostly U.S.-based, because we are most familiar with these programs, and suggest you contact your country's health service for referrals and more updated information. Every effort has been made to ensure that the information we have provided is up to date, but contact information may have changed after publication. By listing these programs, we do not mean to imply that we endorse them, and many may use different approaches from those discussed in this book.

DIAGNOSIS AND TREATMENT

United States

Northeast

CONNECTICUT

Renfrew Center Foundation

MARYLAND

Center for Eating Disorders at Sheppard Pratt

MASSACHUSETTS

Massachusetts General Hospital/Eating Disorders Clinical and Research Program

Boston Children's Hospital
Eating Disorder Program/Adolescent Medicine

NEW HAMPSHIRE

Center for Eating Disorders Management

NEW JERSEY

Eating Disorders Treatment Centers

NEW YORK

New York State Psychiatric Institute/Columbia Center for Eating Disorders

Mount Sinai Eating and Weight Disorders Program
Department of Psychiatry
The Mount Sinai Hospital

PENNSYLVANIA

Renfrew Center Foundation

Center for Overcoming Problem Eating
Western Psychiatric Institute and Clinic
University of Pittsburgh Medical Center

Children's Hospital of Philadelphia/Eating Disorder Services
Division of Adolescent Medicine
Department of Pediatrics
Perelman School of Medicine at the University of Pennsylvania

WASHINGTON, DC

National Medical Center/Eating Disorders Program
Adolescent Medicine/Eating Disorders Program
Children's Hospital

South

LOUISIANA

River Oaks Hospital/Eating Disorders Treatment Center

Resources

NORTH CAROLINA

Duke Center for Eating Disorders
Department of Psychiatry
Duke University

University of North Carolina at Chapel Hill/Eating Disorders Program

Midwest

ILLINOIS

Alexian Brothers Behavioral Health Hospital

University of Chicago Medicine/Eating Disorders Program
Department of Psychiatry
University of Chicago

IOWA

University of Iowa Hospitals and Clinics/
Eating and Weight Disorder Program

MINNESOTA

Emily Program

Children's Hospitals and Clinics of Minnesota/Center for the Treatment of Eating Disorders

Park Nicollet Melrose Center

MISSOURI

McCallum Place

NEBRASKA

Children's Hospital and Medical Center/Eating Disorder Program

NORTH DAKOTA

The Eating Disorders Institute
University of North Dakota

WISCONSIN

Rogers Memorial Hospital/Eating Disorder Services

Southwest

OKLAHOMA

Laureate

TEXAS

Menninger Clinic

University of Texas, Southwestern Medical Center/
Eating Disorders Services Program

West

CALIFORNIA

Center for Discovery

University of California, Los Angeles/Eating Disorders Program
Resnick Neuropsychiatric Hospital at UCLA

Stanford University School of Medicine/Eating Disorders Program for Treatment and Research

University of California, San Diego, School of Medicine/Eating Disorders Center for Treatment and Research

University of California, San Francisco/Eating Disorders Program
UCSF Division of Adolescent and Young Adult Medicine, Department of Pediatrics
Department of Psychiatry, Benioff Children's Hospital

WASHINGTON

Eating and Weight Disorders Program of Seattle

Children's Hospital and Regional Medical Center/
Eating Disorders Program
Department of Child and Adolescent Psychiatry and Behavioral Health

Resources

Canada
BC Children's Hospital/Provincial Specialized Eating Disorders Program for Children and Adolescents

Dalhousie University Medical School/Eating Disorders Clinic
Department of Psychiatry
IWK Health Centre Child and Adolescent Mental Health Program

Hospital for Sick Children/Eating Disorder Program
University of Toronto

Children's Hospital of Eastern Ontario/Eating Disorders Program

McMaster Children's Hospital Eating Disorder Program
Hamilton Health Sciences
Hamilton, Ontario

United Kingdom
Great Ormond Street Hospital for Children NHS Trust

University of London/Eating Disorders Unit
Maudsley Hospital Institute of Psychiatry
Kings College, University of London

Royal Free Hospital

South West London and St. George's Eating Disorders Service
Child and Adolescent Service

Leicester University/Eating Disorders Service
Division of Psychiatry

Alder Hey Children's Hospital Eating Disorder Program
Liverpool, UK

Australia
Children's Hospital at Westmead

Centre for Adolescent Health/Eating Disorders Program
Royal Children's Hospital Melbourne
Centre for Adolescent Health

Centre for Clinical Interventions
Northbridge, Western Australia 6003

New Zealand

Regional Eating Disorders Service
Auckland District Health Board

New Zealand Eating Disorder Clinic
Auckland, NZ

EDUCATION/ADVOCACY/REFERRAL

United States

Academy for Eating Disorders
Phone: 847-498-4274
E-mail: *info@aedweb.org*
Website: *www.aedweb.org*

    The Academy for Eating Disorders is an international transdisciplinary professional organization that promotes excellence in research, treatment, and prevention of eating disorders. Provides education, training, and a forum for collaboration and professional dialogue.

American Academy of Child and Adolescent Psychiatry
Phone: 202-966-7300
Website: *www.aacap.org*

    The mission of AACAP is to promote mentally healthy children, adolescents, and families through research, training, advocacy, prevention, comprehensive diagnosis and treatment, peer support, and collaboration.

Eating Disorder Referral and Information Center
Website: *www.edreferral.com*

    The Eating Disorder Referral and Information Center provides referrals to eating disorder practitioners, treatment facilities, and support groups. Referrals to eating disorder specialists are offered at no charge as a community service.

Eating Disorders Coalition
Washington, DC 20001
Phone: 202-543-9570
Website: *www.eatingdisorderscoalition.org*

The Eating Disorders Coalition for Research, Policy, and Action is a cooperative of professional and advocacy-based organizations committed to federal advocacy on behalf of people with eating disorders, their families, and professionals working with these populations.

National Alliance for Eating Disorders
Phone: 561-841-0900
Helpline: 866-662-1235
Website: *www.allianceforeatingdisorders.com*
The National Alliance for Eating Disorders disseminates educational information to parents and caregivers about the warning signs, dangers, and consequences of anorexia, bulimia, and related disorders.

National Association of Anorexia Nervosa and Associated Disorders
Naperville, IL 60566
Helpline: 630-577-1330
E-mail: *hello@anad.org*
Website: *www.anad.org*
ANAD provides hotline counseling, a national network of free support groups, referrals to health care professionals, and education and prevention programs to promote self-acceptance and healthy lifestyles. All services are free of charge. ANAD also lobbies for state and national health insurance parity and both undertakes and encourages research.

National Eating Disorders Association
New York, NY 10605
Phone: 212-575-6200
E-mail: *info@NationalEatingDisorders.org*
Website: *www.nationaleatingdisorders.org*
The National Eating Disorders Association is the largest not-for-profit organization in the United States working to prevent eating disorders and provide treatment referrals to those suffering from anorexia, bulimia, and binge-eating disorder and those concerned with body image and weight issues.

Society for Adolescent Health and Medicine
Schaumburg, IL 60173
Phone: 847-375-4848
Website: *www.adolescenthealth.org*
A multidisciplinary organization of professionals committed to improving the physical and psychosocial health and well-being of all adolescents.

Canada
ANEB (Anorexia and Bulimia Quebec)
5500 Autoroute Transcandienne Est.
Pointe-Claire, Quebec H9R 1B6
Phone: 514-630-0907
Website: *www.anebquebec.com*

National Eating Disorder Information Centre
Toronto, Ontario M5G 2C4, Canada
Phone: 866-NEDIC-20 (toll free) or 416-340-4156
Website: *www.nedic.ca*
E-mail: *nedic@uhn.on.ca*

This Toronto-based nonprofit organization provides information and resources on eating disorders and weight preoccupation.

United Kingdom
National Centre for Eating Disorders
Phone: 0845 838 2040
Website: *www.eating-disorders.org.uk*

The National Centre for Eating Disorders is an independent organization set up to provide solutions for all eating problems, including binge eating, bulimia, and anorexia. Services include counseling, professional training, and information for students, journalists, and carers. It is the leading organization providing information, help, and support across the United Kingdom, targeted for people whose lives are affected by eating disorders. It aims to positively influence public understanding and policy.

Other International
IAEDP—International Association of Eating Disorders Professionals
Phone: 800-800-8126
Website: *https://iaedpfoundation.com*

The IAEDP aims to provide a high level of professionalism among practitioners who treat those suffering from eating disorders by emphasizing ethical and professional standards, offering education and training in the field, and certifying those who have met professional requirements.

Websites
Beat Eating Disorders: *www.beateatingdisorders.org.uk*
Butterfly Foundation: *www.butterfly.org.au*
Eva Musby: *http://anorexiafamily.com/connecting-child-parent-anorexia*
Families Empowered and Supporting Treatment of Eating Disorders
   (FEAST): *www.feast-ed.org*

Further Reading

American Academy of Pediatrics. (2003). Policy statement: Identifying and treating eating disorders. *Pediatrics, 111,* 204–211.

Andrés-Perpiña, S., Lozano-Serra, E., Puig, O., Lera-Miguel, S., Lázaro, L., & Castro-Fornieles, J. (2011). Clinical and biological correlates of adolescent anorexia nervosa with impaired cognitive profile. *European Child and Adolescent Psychiatry, 50,* 541–549.

Arcelus, J., Mitchell, A., Wales, J., & Nielsen, S. (2011). Mortality rates in patients with anorexia nervosa and other eating disorders. *Archives of General Psychiatry, 68,* 724–731.

Brownell, K. D., & Walsh, B. T. (Eds.). (2017). *Eating Disorders and Obesity: A Comprehensive Handbook* (3rd ed.). New York: Guilford Press.

Bryant-Waugh, R. (2020). *Avoidant/Restrictive Food Intake Disorder: A Guide for Parents and Carers.* New York: Routledge.

Couturier, J., & Lock, J. (2007). Review of medication use for children and adolescents with eating disorders. *Journal of the Canadian Academy of Child and Adolescent Psychiatry, 16,* 173–176.

Crow, S., Peterson, C., Swanson, S., Raymond, N., Specker, S., Eckert, E., & Mitchell, J. (2009). Increased mortality in bulimia nervosa and other eating disorders. *American Journal of Psychiatry, 166,* 1342–1346.

Dalle Grave, R., Conti, M., Sartirana, M., Sermattee, S., & Calugi, S. (2021). Enhanced cognitive behavioral therapy for adolescents with eating disorders: A systematic review of current status and future perspectives. *International Journal of Eating Disorders and Obesity, 3,* 1–11.

Datta, N., Matheson, B., Citron, K., Van Wye, E., & Lock, J. (2023). Evidence based update on psychosocial interventions for eating disorders in children and adolescents. *Journal of Clinical Child and Adolescent Psychology, 52*(2), 159–170.

Fairburn, C. G. (1997). Interpersonal Psychotherapy for Bulimia Nervosa. In D. M. Garner & P. F. Garfinkel (Eds.), *Handbook of Treatment for Eating Disorders* (2nd ed., pp. 278–294). New York: Guilford Press.

Fairburn, C. G. (2008). *Cognitive Behavior Therapy and Eating Disorders.* New York: Guilford Press.

Fairburn, C. G., Cooper, Z., & Shafran, R. (2008). Enhanced Cognitive Behavior Therapy for Eating Disorders ("CBT-E"): An Overview. In C. G. Fairburn, *Cognitive Behavior Therapy and Eating Disorders* (pp. 23–34). New York: Guilford Press.

Gull, W. (1874). Anorexia nervosa (*apepsia hysterica, anorexia hysterica*). *Transactions of the Clinical Society of London, 7,* 222–228.

Hoek, H., & van Hoeken, D. (2003). Review of prevalence and incidence of eating disorders. *International Journal of Eating Disorders, 34,* 383–396.

Keys, A., Brozek, J., & Henschel, A. (1950). *The Biology of Human Starvation*. Minneapolis: University of Minnesota Press.

Lasègue, E. (1883). De l'anorexie hystérique. *Archives Générales de Médecine, 21,* 384–403.

Le Grange, D., Crosby, R., Rathouz, P., & Leventhal, B. (2007). A randomized controlled comparison of family-based treatment and supportive psychotherapy for adolescent bulimia nervosa. *Archives of General Psychiatry, 64,* 1049–1056.

Le Grange, D., Doyle, P., Swanson, S., Ludwig, K., Glunz, C., & Kreipe, R. (2012). Calculation of expected body weight in adolescents with eating disorders. *Pediatrics, 129,* e438–e446.

Le Grange, D., Eckhardt, S., Dalle Grave, R., Crosby, R., Peterson, C., Keery, H., . . . Martell, C. (2020). Enhanced cognitive-behavior therapy and family-based treatment for adolescents with an eating disorder: A non-randomized effectiveness trial. *Psychological Medicine, 52*(13), 1–11.

Le Grange, D., Hughes, E., Court, A., Yeo, M., Crosby, R., & Sawyer, S. (2016). Randomized clinical trial of parent focused therapy and family-based treatment for adolescent anorexia nervosa. *Journal of the American Academy of Child and Adolescent Psychiatry, 55*(8), 683–692.

Le Grange, D., & Lock, J. (2007). *Treating Bulimia in Adolescents: A Family-Based Approach*. New York: Guilford Press.

Le Grange, D., & Lock, J. (Eds.). (2011). *Eating Disorders in Children and Adolescents*. New York: Guilford Press.

Le Grange, D., Lock, J., Agras, W., Bryson, S., & Jo, B. (2015). Randomized clinical trial comparing family based treatment and cognitive behavioral therapy for adolescent bulimia nervosa. *Journal of the American Academy of Child and Adolescent Psychiatry, 54*(11), 886–894.

Le Grange, D., Lock, J., Loeb, K., & Nicholls, D. (2010). Academy for Eating Disorders position paper: The role of the family in eating disorders. *International Journal of Eating Disorders, 43,* 1–5.

Lock, J. (2005). Adjusting cognitive behavioral therapy for adolescent bulimia nervosa: Results of a case series. *American Journal of Psychotherapy, 59,* 267–281.

Lock, J. (2008). Fitting square pegs into round holes: Males with eating disorders. *Journal of Adolescent Health, 44,* 99–100.

Lock, J. (2012). *The Oxford Handbook of Child and Adolescent Eating Disorders: Developmental Perspectives*. New York: Oxford University Press.

Lock, J. (2020). *Adolescent-Focused Therapy for Anorexia Nervosa: A Developmental Approach*. New York: Guilford Press.

Lock, J. (2022). *Family-Based Treatment for Avoidant/Restrictive Food Intake Disorder*. New York: Routledge.

Further Reading

Lock, J., Agras, W. S., Bryson, S., & Kraemer, H. (2005). A comparison of short- and long-term family therapy for adolescent anorexia nervosa. *Journal of the American Academy of Child and Adolescent Psychiatry, 44*, 632–639.

Lock, J., Couturier, J., Matheson, B., Datta, N., Sami, S., Welch, H., . . . John-Carson, N. (2021). Feasibility of conducting a randomized clinical trial comparing family-based treatment via teleconferencing and online guided self-help family-based treatment for adolescent anorexia nervosa. *International Journal of Eating Disorders, 54*(11), 1998–2008.

Lock, J., Le Grange, D., Agras, W. S., Moye, A., Bryson, S., & Jo, B. (2010). Randomized clinical trial comparing family-based treatment to adolescent-focused individual therapy for adolescents with anorexia nervosa. *Archives of General Psychiatry, 67*, 1025–1032.

Lock, J., Le Grange, D., Bohon, C., Matheson, B., & Jo, B. (2024). Who responds to an adaptive treatment for adolescents with anorexia nervosa? Outcomes from a randomized clinical trial. *Journal of the American Academy of Child and Adolescent Psychiatry, 63*(6), 605–614.

Lock, J., Sadeh-Sharvit, S., & L'Insalata, A. (2019). Feasibility of conducting a randomized clinical trial using family-based treatment for avoidant/restrictive food intake disorder. *International Journal of Eating Disorders, 52*, 746–751.

Lock, J., Whyte, A., Matheson, B., & Datta, N. (2024). *Family-Based Treatment for Eating Disorders Piece by Piece: A Practical Guide for Parents*. New York: Routledge.

Loeb, K., Lock, J., Le Grange, D., & Greif, R. (2012). Transdiagnostic theory and application of family-based treatment for youth with eating disorders. *Cognitive and Behavioral Practice, 19*(1), 17–30.

Madden, S., Miskovic-Wheatley, J., Wallis, A., Kohn, M., Lock, J., Le Grange, D. . . . Touyz, S. (2014). A randomized controlled trial of in-patient treatment for anorexia nervosa in medically unstable adolescents. *Psychological Medicine, 44*, 1053–1064.

Safer, D., Couturier, J., & Lock, J. (2007). Dialectical behavior therapy modified for adolescent binge eating disorders: A case report. *Cognitive Behavioral Practice, 14*, 157–167.

Saraf, M. (1998). Holy anorexia and anorexia nervosa: Society and concept of disease. *Pharos, 61*, 2–4.

Silverman, J. (1997). Charcot's comments on the therapeutic role of isolation in the treatment of anorexia nervosa. *International Journal of Eating Disorders, 21*, 295–298.

Swanson, S., Crow, S., Le Grange, D., Swendsen, J., & Merikangas, K. (2011). Prevalence and correlates of eating disorders in adolescents. *Archives of General Psychiatry, 68*, 714–723.

Tchanturia, K., & Lock, J. (2010). Cognitive Remediation Therapy for Eating Disorders: Development, Refinement, and Future Directions. In R. Adan & W. H. Kaye (Eds.), *Behavioral Neurobiology of Eating Disorders* (pp. 269–287). Berlin: Springer-Verlag.

Treasure, J. (1997). *Anorexia Nervosa: A Survival Guide for Families, Friends, and Sufferers*. East Sussex, UK: Psychology Press.

Treasure, J., Schmidt, U., & MacDonald, P. (2010). *The Clinician's Guide to Collaborative Caring in Eating Disorders: The New Maudsley Method*. London: Routledge.

Index

Note. f following a page number indicates a figure.

Abuse, 33, 34
Adolescent-focused therapy (AFT). *See also* Treatment approaches
   anorexia nervosa, 130
   compared to FBT, 134
   overview, 67, 70–71, 136, 139
   parents' roles in, 208–211
Age factors, 205, 241–242. *See also* Developmental factors
Agreement between parents. *See* Disagreements between parents; Parental agreement
Alcohol abuse, 101, 110
All-or-nothing thinking, 108–109. *See also* Cognitive distortions
Anger, 25, 159, 163–164
Anorexia nervosa
   adolescent-focused therapy (AFT) and, 208–209
   body image distortion and, 122
   causation and, 63–64, 74–75
   cognitive-behavioral therapy (CBT) and, 139
   compared to ARFID, 88
   current approaches to treatment and the family's role in, 45–55
   development of, 17–21
   developmental factors, 70–71
   diagnosis and, 5, 21
   early intervention and, 37
   family-based treatment (FBT) and, 57, 58, 133–135, 139
   gender and, 9
   helping your child eat more, 173–178
   helping your child expand food choices, 178–180
   helping your child use exercise appropriately, 181
   historical perspective of, 62–63
   importance placed on not eating or weight loss and, 118–119
   medical complications of, 15–16, 89–93
   medications and, 140–141
   neurotransmitters and, 65–66
   overview, 7, 84–87
   psychological treatments and, 129–131
   thought processes of your child with, 105, 107–126
   warning signs of an eating disorder, 27–30
   working together as a family and, 223
Antidepressants, 101, 140, 141, 142–143. *See also* Medications
Antipsychotics, 101, 140. *See also* Medications
Anxiety
   adolescent development and, 70
   avoidant/restrictive food intake disorder (ARFID), 26–27
   causation and, 65
   challenges related to diagnosis and, 35–36
   current approaches to treatment and the family's role in, 50
   effects of an eating disorder and, 42
   evaluating for an eating disorder and, 34
   family-based treatment (FBT) and, 57
   helping your child prevent binge eating and purging, 183
   knowing when to back off, 192–193
   medications and, 193
   refeeding programs and, 50–51
   regarding food intake, 120–121
Anxiety disorders, 26–27, 33. *See also* Anxiety

Index

Arguments. *See* Conflicts between parents and children; Disagreements between parents; Negotiating with your child
Attention-deficit/hyperactivity disorder, 101
Autism spectrum disorder, 68, 101
Autonomy, 43–44, 48–49, 53, 110–113, 130
Avoidance, 70, 75–76, 86, 100, 207
Avoidant/restrictive food intake disorder (ARFID)
   being available to monitor eating and, 169
   body image distortion and, 122
   causation and, 63
   cognitive-behavioral therapy (CBT) and, 138, 139, 211, 214–215
   denial of an eating disorder diagnosis by a professional and, 249
   denial of by one parent, 228
   development of, 25–27
   diagnosis and, 5
   early intervention and, 3
   effects of an eating disorder and, 45
   family-based treatment (FBT) and, 56, 139
   helping your child eat more, 173–178
   helping your child expand food choices, 178–180
   historical perspective of, 63
   medical complications of, 16–17, 97
   medications and, 142
   overview, 7, 85, 88
   psychological treatments and, 132
   shame and, 124–125
   supporting intensive treatments and, 202
   thought processes of your child with, 104, 105, 115–116, 124–125
   trauma and, 75–76
   warning signs of an eating disorder, 27–30
   working together as a family and, 223

Beauty standards and ideals, 72–74, 188–191. *See also* Body image
Behavioral issues, 33, 34, 65, 110–111
Beliefs, 105–107, 116–120. *See also* Cognitive distortions
Binge eating–purging type of anorexia nervosa, 86–87. *See also* Anorexia nervosa; Binge-eating behavior; Purging behaviors
Binge-eating behavior. *See also* Binge-eating disorder (BED); Bulimia nervosa; Eating behaviors
   anorexia nervosa and, 87
   bulimia nervosa, 87
   cognitive distortions and, 112–113, 123–124
   cognitive-behavioral therapy (CBT) and, 137, 211–215
   depression and, 99–100
   development of an eating disorder and, 21–24
   establishing a pattern of eating and, 171–172
   evaluating for an eating disorder and, 33
   helping your child prevent, 182–185
   intensive treatments and, 143–144
   medical complications of bulimia nervosa, 93–96
   warning signs of an eating disorder, 27
Binge-eating disorder (BED). *See also* Binge-eating behavior
   being available to monitor eating and, 169
   body image distortion and, 122
   causation and, 63
   cognitive-behavioral therapy (CBT) and, 138, 139, 211–215
   denial of by one parent, 228
   denial of the seriousness of, 114–115
   development of, 24–25
   diagnosis and, 5
   dialectical behavior therapy (DBT) and, 219
   family-based treatment (FBT) and, 58
   helping your child use exercise appropriately, 181–182
   historical perspective of, 63
   interpersonal psychotherapy (IPT) and, 138, 215–219
   medical complications of, 16, 96–97
   medications and, 66, 141, 142
   overview, 7, 84–85, 87–88
   psychological treatments and, 132
   thought processes of your child with, 105, 107, 112–113
   warning signs of an eating disorder, 27–30
   working together as a family and, 223
Biological factors, 64–68
Blame. *See also* Causation
   avoiding, 161–165
   current approaches to treatment and the family's role in, 52–53
   disagreements between parents regarding, 230–231
   family-based treatment (FBT) and, 57, 133–134
   parenting practices and, 46–48
   principles of FBT and, 155
   self-blame by parents, 61–63

Blood pressure, 15, 16, 91–92, 97, 201. *See also* Medical risks/health problems
Body checking behavior, 125
Body image
  anorexia nervosa, 86
  beauty standards and ideals, 72–74
  body image distortion, 122–123
  current approaches to treatment and the family's role in, 52
  media influences and, 71–72
  Western cultural ideas of beauty and, 72–74, 188–191
Body mass index, 35, 86. *See also* Weight loss
Body temperature, 15, 91, 201. *See also* Medical risks/health problems
Bone marrow hypoplasia, 92. *See also* Medical risks/health problems
Borderline personality traits, 100. *See also* Personality
Bradycardia, 15, 91, 92. *See also* Medical risks/health problems
Brain activity and changes, 65–66, 92, 93. *See also* Medical risks/health problems
Breakfast, 171–172. *See also* Mealtimes
Breathing, fears related to, 115–116
Bulimia nervosa
  being available to monitor eating and, 169
  body image distortion and, 122
  causation and, 63
  cognitive-behavioral therapy (CBT) and, 137, 139
  control and cognitive distortions and, 112–113
  denial of by one parent, 228
  denial of the seriousness of, 114–115
  development of, 21–24
  diagnosis and, 5
  dialectical behavior therapy (DBT) and, 219
  early intervention and, 37
  evaluating for an eating disorder and, 33
  family-based treatment (FBT) and, 56, 57, 58, 139
  gender and, 9
  helping your child use exercise appropriately, 181–182
  historical perspective of, 63
  importance placed on not eating or weight loss and, 119
  interpersonal psychotherapy (IPT) and, 138, 215–219
  medical complications of, 16, 93–96
  medications and, 66, 141, 142
  neurotransmitters and, 65–66
  overview, 7, 84–85, 87
  psychological treatments and, 131
  shame and, 124
  thought processes of your child with, 105, 107, 124
  warning signs of an eating disorder, 27–30
  working together as a family and, 223

Calorie counting, 28, 33, 178–179. *See also* Dieting
Cardiac problems, 16, 93, 95, 97. *See also* Heart rate; Medical risks/health problems
Causation. *See also* Blame
  avoiding blaming the child or yourself, 161–165
  biological and genetic factors, 64–68
  developmental factors, 69–71
  factors in, 63–76
  family factors, 68–69
  family-based treatment (FBT) and, 133–134
  focusing on treatment rather than, 76–78, 165–185
  principles of FBT and, 155
  self-blame by parents, 61–63
  social and cultural factors, 71–75
  trauma and, 75–76
Changing eating-disordered behaviors. *See also* Consequences for not eating; Eating behaviors; Strategies parents can take
  avoiding blaming the child or yourself and, 161–165
  avoiding debating about eating or weight-related concerns, 185–191
  being available to monitor eating, 166–171
  establishing a pattern of eating, 171–173
  helping your child eat more, 173–178
  helping your child expand food choices, 178–180
  helping your child prevent binge eating and purging, 182–185
  helping your child use exercise appropriately, 180–182
  making a top priority of, 165–166
  working together as a family, 157–161
  working with experts and, 156–157
Child characteristics, 41–45, 42*f*. *See also* Personality
Choices, 174–175, 178–180, 186–187, 241–243
Choking, fear of, 25–27, 115–116. *See also* Avoidant/restrictive food intake disorder (ARFID)

Index

Clinical depression. *See* Depression
Clinicians, 58–59, 147, 155, 198. *See also* Experts; Professional help
Clothes shopping, 187
Cognitive distortions
  avoiding debating about eating or weight-related concerns, 185–186
  body checking and repeated weighing, 125
  body image distortion, 122–123
  control and, 110–113
  denial of the seriousness of an eating disorder, 113–116
  helping your child eat more, 177–178
  helping your child expand food choices, 179–180
  importance placed on not eating or weight loss and, 118–120
  intentions and promises and, 126
  overview, 104–105, 107–126, 137
  perfectionism and, 108–110
  pride and, 124–125
  purging and, 123–124
  regarding food intake, 120–121, 177–178
  separating the illness from the adolescent and, 116–118, 126–127
  understanding the thought processes of your child with an eating disorder and, 105–107
  working together as a family and, 159
Cognitive remediation therapy (CRT), 219–220
Cognitive-behavioral therapy (CBT). *See also* Treatment approaches
  anorexia nervosa, 130–131
  avoidant/restrictive food intake disorder (ARFID), 132
  binge-eating disorder (BED), 132
  bulimia nervosa, 131
  medications in addition to, 142–143
  overview, 67, 137–138, 139
  parents' roles in supporting, 211–215
Communication, 207, 256–257. *See also* Negotiating with your child
Comorbidity, 33, 97–102, 140–141. *See also* Psychological illnesses
Complexity of eating disorders. *See also* Anorexia nervosa; Avoidant/restrictive food intake disorder (ARFID); Binge-eating disorder (BED); Bulimia nervosa; Understanding eating disorders
  denial of the seriousness of an eating disorder and, 113–116
  how eating disorders slip through, 224–225

medical complications and, 89–97
other psychological illnesses and, 97–102
overview, 83–97, 102
thinking distortions and, 104–105
treatment and, 146–147
Confidentiality, 34, 198, 209–210
Conflict between parents. *See* Disagreements between parents; Parental agreement
Conflicts between parents and children. *See also* Negotiating with your child; Parent–child relationship
  avoiding debating about eating or weight-related concerns, 185–191
  current approaches to treatment and the family's role in, 53–54
  divide-and-conquer scenarios and, 225–239
  effects of an eating disorder and, 41–45, 42*f*
  general family therapy and, 207
  helping your child expand food choices, 180
  intentions and promises and, 126
  principles of FBT and, 155
  regarding food intake, 120–121, 176–178
  separating the illness from the adolescent and, 116–118
  working together as a family, 157–161
Consequences for not eating, 162–163, 174–176. *See also* Changing eating-disordered behaviors
Control, 49–51, 110–113
Cultural factors, 7–8, 52, 71–75, 188–191

Day-patient treatment, 143, 200–206. *See also* Intensive treatments; Treatment approaches
Death, 15, 16, 115–116. *See also* Medical risks/health problems
Debating with your child. *See* Conflicts between parents and children; Negotiating with your child
Decision making, 241–243. *See also* Choices
Dehydration, 16, 91, 95. *See also* Medical risks/health problems
Denial of the seriousness of an eating disorder, 113–116, 154, 227–229, 247–249. *See also* Cognitive distortions
Depression
  binge-eating disorder (BED), 25
  challenges related to diagnosis and, 35–36
  evaluating for an eating disorder and, 33, 34

Depression (*continued*)
  medications and, 141, 193
  overview, 99–100
  risks associated with eating disorders and, 15
Development of an eating disorder
  anorexia nervosa, 17–21
  avoidant/restrictive food intake disorder (ARFID), 25–27
  binge-eating disorder (BED), 24–25
  bulimia nervosa, 21–24
  focusing on treatment rather than causation and, 76–78
  overview, 17–27
  warning signs of an eating disorder, 27–30
Developmental factors, 5, 34, 43–44, 49, 69–71. *See also* Development of an eating disorder
Diabetes, 16, 97. *See also* Medical risks/health problems
Diagnosis
  anorexia nervosa, 21, 86
  avoidant/restrictive food intake disorder (ARFID), 88
  bulimia nervosa, 87
  challenges related to, 35–37
  denial of an eating disorder diagnosis by a professional and, 247–249
  denial of by one parent, 227–229
  historical perspective of, 62–63
  overview, 5
Diagnostic and Statistical Manual of Mental Disorders (DSM-5)
  anorexia nervosa, 86
  avoidant/restrictive food intake disorder (ARFID), 88
  challenges related to diagnosis and, 36
  development of an eating disorder and, 21
  historical perspective of eating disorders and, 63
  overview, 5
Dialectical behavior therapy (DBT), 131, 132, 219. *See also* Treatment approaches
Diet pill use, 20, 27, 33
Dieting. *See also* Food restriction
  anorexia nervosa, 19–21, 86–87
  binge-eating disorder (BED), 25
  bulimia nervosa, 21–24, 87
  calorie counting, 28, 33, 178–179
  cognitive distortions and, 108–110
  denial of the seriousness of an eating disorder and, 114
  development of an eating disorder and, 19–24, 25
  evaluating for an eating disorder and, 33
  helping your child expand food choices, 178–179
  importance placed on not eating or weight loss and, 118–120
  warning signs of an eating disorder, 27–30
  wealth factors and, 74–75
Dietitians, 35, 50–51. *See also* Professional help
Digital media. *See* Media influences
Dinner, 171–172. *See also* Mealtimes
Disagreements between parents. *See also* Parental agreement
  blame and, 230–231
  denial by one parent, 227–229
  divide-and-conquer scenarios and, 225–239
  divorce or other circumstances and, 234–236
  how eating disorders slip through, 224–225
  only one parent recognizing the urgency of treatment, 225–227
  regarding how the eating disorder is addressed, 229–230, 231–233
  regarding weight gain, 233–234
  when one parent feels defeated, 236–238
  when parents take turns siding with the adolescent/eating disorder, 238–239
Distorted thinking. *See* Cognitive distortions
Distraction, 165–185
Divorce, 234–236. *See also* Single-parent families
Dizziness, 33
Dopamine, 65–66
Drinks, 33, 180
Drive, 20, 65
Drug abuse, 101, 110

Early intervention. *See also* Evaluation for an eating disorder; Professional help; Treatment approaches; Urgency of obtaining treatment
  focusing on treatment rather than causation and, 76–78
  identifying problems and, 15–17
  importance of, 37, 102, 146
  overview, 3
  urgency and, 6–7
Eating behaviors. *See also* Binge-eating behavior; Changing eating-disordered behaviors; Food restriction
  anorexia nervosa, 86
  avoiding debating about eating or weight-related concerns, 185–191

Index

cognitive distortions and, 120–121
cognitive-behavioral therapy (CBT) and, 137, 213–215
development of an eating disorder and, 20–27
establishing a pattern of eating, 171–173
evaluating for an eating disorder and, 32–34
helping your child eat more, 173–178
helping your child expand food choices, 178–180
helping your child prevent binge eating and purging, 182–185
making changing disordered eating a top priority, 165–166
overeating episodes, 87, 182–185
warning signs of an eating disorder, 27
working together as a family and, 159
Eating disorders, becoming informed regarding. *See* Complexity of eating disorders; Understanding eating disorders
Effects of an eating disorder, 41–45, 42*f*. *See also* Medical risks/health problems
Ego-syntonic illness, 89–90, 114–115
Electrical brain activity. *See* Brain activity and changes
Emotions
causation and, 65
development of an eating disorder and, 20–21, 24, 25
effects of an eating disorder on, 41
separating the illness from the adolescent and, 116–118
working together as a family and, 159
Empowerment, parental, 57–58, 59. *See also* Parent's involvement in treatment
Enamel loss, 16, 96. *See also* Medical risks/health problems
Enhanced cognitive-behavioral therapy (CBT-E), 67, 130–131. *See also* Cognitive-behavioral therapy (CBT)
Evaluation for an eating disorder. *See also* Early intervention; Professional help
challenges related to diagnosis and, 35–37
getting your child to have an evaluation, 30–31
overview, 28–30
sharing your perspectives, 197–198
what to expect from, 32–35
whom and what to look for in, 31–35
Exercise
anorexia nervosa, 86
development of an eating disorder and, 20
evaluating for an eating disorder and, 33

helping your child use appropriately, 180–182
purging and, 185
warning signs of an eating disorder, 27
Expectations, 155, 174, 176
Experts. *See also* Clinicians; Professional help
being told that they "tried everything," 258–259
communication from professionals and, 256–257
conflicting advice from, 253–257
denial of an eating disorder diagnosis by, 247–249
disagreeing with the advice from, 251–253
exclusion of parents by professionals, 249–250
finding, 259–261
overview, 29–30
too many professionals involved in care, 257–258
working with, 156–157, 245–261
Externalizing the illness. *See* Separating the illness from the adolescent
Extracurricular activities, 20, 108, 170, 181–182

Fainting, 16, 28, 33
Family factors, 33, 68–69, 206–208, 209–210. *See also* Parental agreement
Family involvement, 157–161, 169, 171–173. *See also* Parent's involvement in treatment
Family therapy, 68–69, 206–208. *See also* Family-based treatment (FBT); Treatment approaches
Family therapy for anorexia nervosa (FT-AN), 133–134. *See also* Family-based treatment (FBT)
Family-based treatment (FBT). *See also* Strategies parents can take; Treatment approaches
anorexia nervosa, 129–130
avoidant/restrictive food intake disorder (ARFID), 132
binge-eating disorder (BED), 132
bulimia nervosa, 131
intensive treatments and, 145
overview, 3–4, 55–59, 127, 132–135, 139, 154, 195–196, 206
principles of, 155–156
Fasting behaviors, 27, 33
Fear, 25–27, 115–116, 171–173
Feminist perspectives, 73–74
Fluid intake, 33, 180

Focusing on the disordered eating
  behaviors and beliefs, 165–185. *See
  also* Changing eating-disordered
  behaviors; Separating the illness from
  the adolescent
Follow-up care, 202
Food restriction. *See also* Dieting; Eating
  behaviors
  anorexia nervosa, 86–87
  cognitive distortions and, 107, 108–110,
    120–121
  current approaches to treatment and
    the family's role in, 50
  development of an eating disorder and,
    20–21
  establishing a pattern of eating and,
    171–173
  evaluating for an eating disorder and,
    33
  helping your child eat more, 173–178
  helping your child prevent binge eating
    and purging, 183
  importance placed on not eating or
    weight loss and, 118–120
Friendships. *See* Peer relationships

Gastrointestinal difficulties, 93, 96. *See
  also* Medical risks/health problems
Gender, 9, 74, 205
Genetic factors, 54–68
Grief, 215–216
Grocery shopping, 186–187
Guided self-help (GSH) delivery of FBT,
  129, 134–135. *See also* Family-based
  treatment (FBT)
Guilt, 57–58, 63–64, 120–121, 164–165,
  183

Hair changes, 15, 92. *See also* Medical
  risks/health problems
Health problems. *See* Medical risks/health
  problems; Risks associated with eating
  disorders
Heart disease/problems. *See* Cardiac
  problems; Medical risks/health
  problems
Heart rate, 15, 92, 201. *See also* Cardiac
  problems; Medical risks/health
  problems
Historical perspective of eating disorders,
  62–63
Hormone changes, 92. *See also* Medical
  risks/health problems
Hospital programs, 45–46, 50–52,
  143–146, 200–206. *See also* Intensive
  treatments; Residential treatment;
  Treatment approaches

Hypertension. *See* Blood pressure;
  Medical risks/health problems
Hypokalemia. *See* Potassium depletion
Hypotension. *See* Blood pressure; Medical
  risks/health problems
Hypothermia. *See* Body temperature;
  Medical risks/health problems

Identifying problems. *See also* Symptoms
  of eating disorders; Warning signs of
  an eating disorder
  anorexia nervosa, 17–21
  avoidant/restrictive food intake
    disorder (ARFID), 25–27
  binge-eating disorder (BED), 24–25
  bulimia nervosa, 21–24
  development of an eating disorder and,
    17–27
  overview, 15–17, 27–30
Identity
  adolescent development and, 70
  causation and, 67
  current approaches to treatment and
    the family's role in, 46–48
  effects of an eating disorder and, 41–45,
    42f
  peer relationships and, 188–189
  Western cultural ideas of beauty and,
    72–74
Independence
  control and cognitive distortions and,
    110–113
  current approaches to treatment and
    the family's role in, 48–49
  effects of an eating disorder and, 43–44, 49
  general family therapy and, 207
  intensive treatments and, 144
  involving the child in decision making
    prematurely, 241–242
Individual therapy, 47–53, 135–136, 193,
  208–211. *See also* Adolescent-focused
  therapy (AFT); Cognitive-behavioral
  therapy (CBT); Interpersonal
  psychotherapy (IPT); Outpatient
  treatments; Psychodynamic
  psychotherapy; Treatment approaches
Inpatient treatment, 50–52, 143–146. *See
  also* Hospital programs; Intensive
  treatments
Insight-oriented therapies, 144
Intensive parent coaching (IPC), 135
Intensive psychotherapy, 135–136
Intensive treatments, 143–146, 196–199,
  200–206, 222–223. *See also* Day-
  patient treatment; Hospital programs;
  Inpatient treatment; Residential
  treatment; Treatment approaches

Index

Interpersonal deficits, 215–216. *See also* Relationships
Interpersonal psychotherapy (IPT), 131, 132, 138, 215–219. *See also* Treatment approaches
Involvement of parents in treatment. *See* Parent's involvement in treatment

Laboratory tests, 28–29, 96
Laxative use, 16, 20, 27, 33, 184–185. *See also* Purging behaviors
Learning about eating disorders. *See* Complexity of eating disorders; Understanding eating disorders
Leave from work, 166–171
Lunch, 167–169, 171–172, 191–192. *See also* Mealtimes

Malnutrition, 91, 105–107, 173–178, 200–202. *See also* Medical risks/health problems
Maudsley Approach, 133. *See also* Family-based treatment (FBT)
Mealtimes
  being available to monitor eating and, 166–171
  establishing a pattern of eating, 171–173
  helping your child eat more, 173–178
  helping your child prevent binge eating and purging, 182–183
  knowing when to back off, 191–192
  skipping meals, 27, 33, 171–172
  supporting intensive treatments and, 204, 205
Media influences, 27, 71–72, 74, 188–191
Medical evaluation, 28–29, 96
Medical risks/health problems. *See also* Risks associated with eating disorders
  anorexia nervosa and, 89–93
  avoidant/restrictive food intake disorder (ARFID), 97
  binge-eating disorder (BED), 96–97
  bulimia nervosa, 93–96
  denial of the seriousness of an eating disorder and, 113–116
  evaluating for an eating disorder and, 33
  laxative use and, 184–185
  medications and, 140–141
  overview, 15–17, 28–29, 33
  purging and, 184
  supporting intensive treatments and, 200–202
  treatment and, 147
Medications, 65–66, 101, 140–141, 142–143, 193. *See also* Treatment approaches

Menstruation
  anorexia nervosa and, 91
  effects of an eating disorder and, 49
  evaluating for an eating disorder and, 28, 33
  onset of, 19, 21, 33
  risks associated with eating disorders and, 15–16
  warning signs of an eating disorder, 27
Mental distortions, 106. *See also* Cognitive distortions
Mental illness, 75–76
Monitoring eating, 166–171, 182–183, 191–192, 212–215. *See also* Strategies parents can take
Multifamily groups, 129, 133–134, 219. *See also* Family-based treatment (FBT)

Negotiating with your child. *See also* Conflicts between parents and children; Parent–child relationship; Resistance
  helping your child expand food choices, 180
  intentions and promises and, 126
  principles of FBT and, 155
  regarding food intake, 120–121
  separating the illness from the adolescent and, 118
Neurodevelopmental disorders, 101
Neurotransmitters, 65–66, 75
Nutritional counseling, 139. *See also* Treatment approaches

Obesity, 16, 96–97. *See also* Medical risks/health problems
Obsessive–compulsive disorder, 33, 99
Online delivery of FBT, 129, 135, 260. *See also* Family-based treatment (FBT)
Oppositional defiant disorder, 101
Outpatient treatments, 129–143, 146–147, 222–223. *See also* Individual therapy; Treatment approaches
Overeating episodes, 87, 182–185. *See also* Binge-eating behavior; Eating behaviors

Parent education meetings, 204. *See also* Understanding eating disorders
Parent support groups and therapy, 204
Parental agreement. *See also* Disagreements between parents; Strategies parents can take
  being available to monitor eating and, 167
  divide-and-conquer scenarios and, 225–239

Parental agreement (*continued*)
  divorce or other circumstances and, 234–236
  evaluating for an eating disorder and, 30–31
  helping your child eat more, 176
  how eating disorders slip through, 224–225
  importance of, 243
  involving the child in decision making prematurely, 241–243
  overview, 222–224
  separating the illness from the adolescent and, 239–241
  staying on the right page and, 239–243
  supporting intensive treatments and, 196–197
  when one parent feels defeated, 236–238
  working together as a family and, 157–161
Parental self-care, 155, 193
Parent–child relationship. *See also* Conflicts between parents and children
  current approaches to treatment and the family's role in, 46, 52–54
  effects of an eating disorder and, 41–45, 42*f*, 49
  separating the illness from the adolescent and, 116–118
"Parentectomy," 46, 50–52
Parent-focused therapy (PFT), 129–130. *See also* Family-based treatment (FBT)
Parenting practices
  adolescent-focused therapy (AFT) and, 209–210
  current approaches to treatment and the family's role in, 46–48, 52–54
  disagreements between parents regarding, 229–230, 231–233
  involving the child in decision making prematurely, 242
  self-blame by parents, 61–63
Parent's involvement in treatment. *See also* Changing eating-disordered behaviors; Family-based treatment (FBT); Strategies parents can take
  assessing progress and, 198–199
  cognitive distortions and, 127
  cognitive remediation therapy (CRT) and, 219–220
  cognitive-behavioral therapy (CBT) and, 211–215
  current approaches to treatment and, 45–55
  dialectical behavior therapy (DBT) and, 219
  disagreements between parents regarding, 229–230
  evaluating for an eating disorder and, 34
  exclusion of parents by professionals, 249–250
  experts and, 156–157
  family-based treatment (FBT) and, 55–59
  general family therapy and, 206–208
  importance of, 3–4, 260
  individual therapy approaches and, 47–50, 208–211
  intensive treatments and, 196–199, 200–206
  interpersonal psychotherapy (IPT) and, 215–219
  knowing when to back off, 191–193
  overview, 2–3, 5–6, 8, 39–41, 146–147, 153–154, 195–196, 261
  principles of FBT and, 155–156
  sharing your perspectives, 197–198
  traditional approach to, 2, 3
  ways of, 7–8
  when you're not in charge of treatment, 200–220
Pediatricians, 28–30, 247–249. *See also* Professional help
Peer relationships. *See also* Relationships
  being available to monitor eating and, 170
  development of an eating disorder and, 19
  effects of an eating disorder and, 49
  evaluating for an eating disorder and, 33, 34
  influences of the media and, 188–189
  knowing when to back off, 192
  supportive friendships and, 187–188
  warning signs of an eating disorder, 28
Perfectionism, 20, 41–43, 65, 108–110
Performance, 42–43, 73
Personality
  causation and, 65
  development of an eating disorder and, 20
  effects of an eating disorder on, 41–45, 42*f*
  overview, 100
  wealth factors and, 74–75
  working together as a family and, 159
Personality disorders, 33
Pharmacology. *See* Medications
Physical abuse, 33, 34

Index

Physicians, 28–30, 247–249. *See also* Professional help
Picky eating, 25–27, 47, 116. *See also* Avoidant/restrictive food intake disorder (ARFID)
Posttraumatic stress disorder (PTSD), 101
Potassium depletion, 15, 16, 94–95. *See also* Medical risks/health problems
Pride, 109–110, 114, 124–125
Privacy, 34, 44–45
Pro-eating disorder websites, 27, 190–191
Professional help. *See also* Clinicians; Early intervention; Evaluation for an eating disorder; Experts; Treatment approaches
  assessing progress and, 198–199
  being told that they "tried everything," 258–259
  challenges related to diagnosis and, 35–37
  communication from professionals and, 256–257
  conflicting advice from experts, 253–257
  contact with providers and, 198
  evaluating for an eating disorder and, 28–35
  finding, 259–261
  having a backup plan and, 199
  obtaining, 30–35
  supporting intensive treatments and, 196–199
  too many professionals involved in care, 257–258
  whom and what to look for in, 31–35
  working with experts and, 245–261
Progress assessment, 198–199, 214, 219
Promises, 126. *See also* Negotiating with your child
Psychiatric illnesses. *See* Psychological illnesses
Psychiatric medications. *See* Medications
Psychodynamic psychotherapy, 66–67, 68–69, 135–136, 208–211. *See also* Treatment approaches
Psychological illnesses. *See also* Anxiety; Depression
  in addition to eating disorders, 97–102
  causation and, 62–63
  medications and, 140–141, 193
  overview, 33, 193
  separating the illness from the adolescent and, 126–127
Psychological treatments, 129–139, 143–146. *See also* Adolescent-focused therapy (AFT); Cognitive-behavioral therapy (CBT); Family-based treatment (FBT); Treatment approaches
Punishment, 175. *See also* Consequences for not eating
Purging behaviors. *See also* Vomiting
  anorexia nervosa and, 87
  avoiding blaming the child or yourself and, 163–164
  bulimia nervosa, 87
  cognitive distortions and, 123–124
  cognitive-behavioral therapy (CBT) and, 137, 211–215
  control and cognitive distortions and, 112–113
  depression and, 99–100
  development of an eating disorder and, 21–24
  evaluating for an eating disorder and, 33
  helping your child prevent, 182–185
  intensive treatments and, 143–144
  medical complications of bulimia nervosa, 93–96
  overview, 183–184
  purgatives use, 16, 33
  warning signs of an eating disorder, 27

Refeeding programs, 50–52, 179. *See also* Treatment approaches; Weight restoration
Relationships. *See also* Conflicts between parents and children; Parent–child relationship; Peer relationships
  avoidant personality traits and, 100
  evaluating for an eating disorder and, 33
  influences of the media and, 188–189
  risks associated with eating disorders and, 16
  separating the illness from the adolescent and, 116–118
  supportive friendships and, 187–188
Residential treatment, 45–46, 143–146, 200–206. *See also* Hospital programs; Intensive treatments; Treatment approaches
Resistance, 157–162, 176–180. *See also* Conflicts between parents and children
Restoration of weight. *See* Weight restoration
Restricting type of anorexia nervosa, 86–87. *See also* Anorexia nervosa; Dieting; Food restriction
Restriction, food. *See* Dieting; Food restriction

Risk factors. *See* Causation
Risks associated with eating disorders, 15–17, 113–116. *See also* Medical risks/health problems
Role disputes or transitions, 215–218
Role of family in treatment, 45–55. *See also* Family-based treatment (FBT); Parent's involvement in treatment
Rules, 118–120, 179–180, 183, 186–187

Schedules, 166–171, 172, 192, 199
School attendance, 88, 192, 199
School lunches, 167–169. *See also* Mealtimes
Self-blame, 61–63, 64, 161–165. *See also* Blame
Self-care, parental, 155, 193
Self-esteem, 73, 109
Self-injury, 131
Self-monitoring, 212–214
Self-worth, 73, 87
Separating the illness from the adolescent
  avoiding blaming the child or yourself and, 161–165
  disagreeing with the advice from experts and, 253
  focusing on the disorder rather than the whys, 165–185
  helping your child eat more, 175
  overview, 116–118, 126–127
  parental agreement and, 239–241
  strategies parents can take and, 155
Serotonin, 65–66
Sexual abuse, 34, 75. *See also* Abuse
Sexuality, 67, 70
Shame
  binge-eating disorder (BED), 25
  bulimia nervosa and, 24
  cognitive distortions and, 124–125
  denial of the seriousness of an eating disorder and, 114–115
  family-based treatment (FBT) and, 58
  helping your child prevent binge eating and purging, 183
Shoplifting, 185
Shopping, 186–187
Siblings, 160–161, 169–171
Single-parent families, 215–216, 218, 225, 234–236
Skin, 15, 92. *See also* Medical risks/health problems
Skipping meals, 27, 33, 171–172. *See also* Dieting; Eating behaviors; Food restriction; Mealtimes
Snacks, 171–172, 191–192. *See also* Mealtimes
Social factors, 20, 25, 71–75, 192–193

Social media. *See* Media influences
Specialists, 29–30. *See also* Experts; Professional help
Sports, 20, 108, 170, 181–182
Starvation, 90–91, 99, 106–107, 120–121. *See also* Malnutrition; Medical risks/health problems; Weight loss
Strategies parents can take. *See also* Changing eating-disordered behaviors; Family-based treatment (FBT); Parental agreement; Parent's involvement in treatment
  avoiding blaming the child or yourself, 161–165
  avoiding debating about eating or weight-related concerns, 185–191
  being available to monitor eating, 166–171
  establishing a pattern of eating, 171–173
  helping your child eat more, 173–178
  helping your child expand food choices, 178–180
  helping your child prevent binge eating and purging, 182–185
  helping your child use exercise appropriately, 180–182
  knowing when to back off, 191–193
  making changing disordered eating a top priority, 165–166
  self-care and, 155, 193
  supporting intensive treatments and, 196–199
  working together as a family, 157–161
  working with experts and, 156–157
Structural family therapy for anorexia, 69. *See also* Family therapy; Treatment approaches
Substance abuse, 101, 110
Suicidal ideation, 131
Support groups and therapy for parents, 204
Symptoms of eating disorders. *See also* Identifying problems; Warning signs of an eating disorder
  assessing progress and, 198–199
  denial of the seriousness of an eating disorder and, 113–116
  effects of an eating disorder and, 41–45, 42*f*
  family-based treatment (FBT) and, 56
  focusing on treatment rather than causation and, 76–78
  treatment and, 129
Systemic family therapy, 134. *See also* Family-based treatment (FBT); Treatment approaches

Index

Temperature, body. *See* Body temperature; Medical risks/health problems
Therapists, 147, 155, 198. *See also* Experts; Professional help
Thinking style, 67–68. *See also* Cognitive distortions
Tooth enamel, 16, 96. *See also* Medical risks/health problems
Trauma, 33, 34, 75–76
Travel, 16, 172–173
Treatment, parent's involvement in. *See* Parent's involvement in treatment
Treatment approaches. *See also* Adolescent-focused therapy (AFT); Changing eating-disordered behaviors; Cognitive-behavioral therapy (CBT); Early intervention; Family-based treatment (FBT); Hospital programs; Individual therapy; Intensive treatments; Medications; Outpatient treatments; Parent's involvement in treatment; Professional help; Residential treatment
  causation and, 63–64
  cognitive distortions and, 127
  current approaches to, 45–55
  disagreeing with the advice from experts regarding, 251–253
  disagreements between parents regarding, 225–227
  focusing on treatment rather than causation and, 76–78
  overview, 128–129, 146–147, 153–154
  working with experts and, 246
Treatment team, 246, 253–258, 259–261

Understanding eating disorders. *See also* Anorexia nervosa; Avoidant/restrictive food intake disorder (ARFID); Binge-eating disorder (BED); Bulimia nervosa; Complexity of eating disorders
  causation and, 61–63
  family-based treatment (FBT) and, 57
  medical complications of eating disorders, 89–97
  other psychological illnesses and, 97–102
  overview, 83–84
  psychological and medical components, 84–97
  supporting intensive treatments and, 197, 204
  thought processes of your child with an eating disorder, 105–126

Unity between parents. *See* Parental agreement
Urgency of obtaining treatment. *See also* Early intervention
  disagreements between parents regarding, 225–227
  evaluating for an eating disorder and, 28–29
  focusing on treatment rather than causation and, 76–78
  overview, 6–7, 37, 154, 166–167

Vegetarianism, 27
Videoconference delivery of treatments, 129, 135, 260
Vomiting, 16, 20, 21–24, 123–124. *See also* Purging behaviors
Vomiting, fear of, 25–27. *See also* Avoidant/restrictive food intake disorder (ARFID)

Warning signs of an eating disorder, 27–30, 67–68, 102. *See also* Identifying problems; Symptoms of eating disorders
Wealth factors, 74–75
Websites that are pro-eating disorders, 27, 190–191
Weighing, 125, 186
Weight concerns, 20, 33, 52, 122–123, 185–191. *See also* Dieting
Weight loss. *See also* Body mass index
  anorexia nervosa and, 86, 91
  denial of the seriousness of an eating disorder and, 114
  evaluating for an eating disorder and, 28
  importance placed on not eating or weight loss and, 118–120
  risks associated with eating disorders and, 15–16
  supporting intensive treatments and, 200–206
  warning signs of an eating disorder, 27
Weight restoration, 112, 143–144, 173–178, 200–206, 233–234. *See also* Refeeding programs
Western cultural ideas of beauty, 72–74, 188–191. *See also* Body image; Cultural factors
Working together as a family, 222–224, 225–239. *See also* Parental agreement; Parent's involvement in treatment

About the Authors

James Lock, MD, PhD, is the Eric Rothenberg, MD, Professor of Child Psychiatry and Pediatrics at Stanford University and Director of the Stanford Child and Adolescent Eating Disorders Program. Dr. Lock is committed to providing evidence-based treatments to children, adolescents, and their families. He is a Distinguished Fellow of the American Psychiatric Association and the American Academy of Child and Adolescent Psychiatry, and a recipient of the Agnes Purcell McGavin Award for Distinguished Career Achievement in Child and Adolescent Psychiatry from the American Psychiatric Association, the Price Family Foundation Award for Research Excellence from the National Eating Disorders Association, the Leadership Award in Research from the Academy of Eating Disorders, and Early and Mid-Career Development Awards from the National Institute of Mental Health.

Daniel Le Grange, PhD, is Benioff UCSF Professor in Children's Health in the Department of Psychiatry and UCSF Weill Institute for Neurosciences and Director of the Eating Disorders Program at the University of California, San Francisco. He is Emeritus Professor at the University of Chicago, where he was Director of the Eating Disorders Program until 2014. Dr. Le Grange was a member of the team at the Maudsley Hospital in London that developed family-based treatment for anorexia nervosa. Over his career, he has treated numerous adolescents and families struggling with eating disorders. He is a recipient of the Leadership Award in Research from the Academy of Eating Disorders and an Early Career Development Award from the National Institute of Mental Health.